Quick F

Easy Fasting Instructions
For The 1 to 14 Day Fast

Special thanks

... to my wife, Simone,
who understood why I fasted and brought dinner to the
office during the long night hours of research and writ-
ing when I was not fasting.
... to my proofreaders, Lee Bliss and Traci Bronner,
for their expertise in making technical things clear and
easy to read.
... to Dr. Stephen Tates,
for his knowledge of naturopathic medicine, proofread-
ing, suggestions, support and advice taken from many
years of fasting and supervising patient fasts.
... to my mother, Robbie Bronner,
for encouraging me to study to insure my safety.
... to my late father, Dr. Nathaniel Hawthorne Bronner, Sr.,
for my earthly guidance and for pointing to the path of
health in mind, body and spirit.
... and foremost praise to the Divine Creator,
for directing and protecting me along this path.

Graphic Layout & Design by IN-Line Graphic Solutions

Quick Fasting

Easy Fasting Instructions
For The 1 To 14 Day Fast

Nathaniel Hawthorne Bronner, Jr.

1 gallon = 128 ozs
= 16 glasses
(8 oz)

7TH PRINTING

Century Systems
Atlanta, GA
©1995-2000 All Rights Reserved
ISBN 0-9631075-1-8

This book is available on the world wide web in its entirety at
http://www.1800thewoman.com

10   9   8   7

Contents

[handwritten annotations: "MIRACLE OIL" next to item 10; "22" next to item 11; "12 - 16 8oz glasses distilled water + 1 lemon per gallon" next to item 12]

This book is written for anyone who wishes to fast from one to fourteen days.

Fasts lasting 21 days or more, should be conducted under a doctor's professional supervision or with personalized instructions from a natural health professional. (See Chapter 7, Consulting A Doctor).

Persons on medication or with serious diseases such as diabetes, ulcers, heart disease, kidney or liver malfunction, etc. should consult a doctor before attempting any type of fast.

Pregnant or nursing women should not fast without professional advice.

Be prepared for <u>QUICK FASTING</u> to change your life for the better, just open your mind to the information presented here.

Introduction

Fasting is powerful. Fasting can cure your body. Fasting can open spiritual doors. Fasting can help you attain mastery over self. Fasting can also hurt you if you don't know what you're doing. Few people know how to fast. It's not as simple as it seems. Any endeavor requires knowledge to get the maximum benefit. Would you buy a tennis racket or golf clubs without eventually getting some instructions on how to use them? Would you buy a weight set, and without any prior experience, just start throwing weights up in the air? There are many wrong ways to attempt to do a right thing. With something as powerful as fasting, you should know more about it and how to do it properly because it involves much more than just not eating.

Why should I fast? How long should I fast? Is fasting a good way to lose weight? Should I work while I fast? Can fasting hurt me? Am I too skinny to fast? Am I too fat to fast? How do I prepare for a fast? What is a quick way to tell if my body is in condition for a fast? Do I exercise while I fast? Can I have sex while I fast? These are just a few of the questions this book will answer.

We spend much time figuring out what to eat but when we decide to stop eating, we don't have the proper knowledge to get the most out of our fast. Often, instead of the fast benefiting our bodies, it does us harm because of our lack of knowledge. Proper knowledge can turn a potentially harmful experience into a blessing that is beyond price.

Observing religious beliefs, seeking God, and maintaining and/or improving one's health are the major reasons for fasting. Fasting is recognized by every major religion. The benefits of fasting are universally recognized for spiritual development but how many times have you heard anyone tell you how to properly conduct your fast?

I am a Christian, a follower of Jesus, the Christ. I have been in many churches where the congregation fasted, but not once was anyone told anything about how to fast other than to simply **STOP EATING!**

There is more to a fast than that ... MUCH MORE!

Chapter 1

What is Fasting

Fasting is the abstaining from **ALL FOOD.** Fasting means taking in nothing but **WATER.** NO JUICE, NO FRUIT, NO TEAS, **NOTHING BUT WATER.**

Often people will make the comment, "I'm fasting, I just have my coffee in the morning and a sandwich in the afternoon." That is not fasting. Fasting in its **strictest sense** is the total abstinence from anything considered food, and that's anything but water. There are modified fasts such as a juice fast, i.e., consuming nothing but fruit and/or vegetable juices or a fruit fast, consuming nothing but raw fruits.

There are other such fasts that abstain from everything EXCEPT the item that precedes the word "fast". For example, a grapefruit fast, is abstaining from everything except grapefruits. Many health enthusiasts, for particular reasons, may place individuals on particular types of fasts restricting them to one or a group of foods (usually fruits or teas), for healing purposes.

This book deals with the true fast, NOTHING BUT WATER. When I use the word fast, just as in the scriptures, I mean nothing but water.

Many ask, "If I'm on a fast can I have a little piece of fruit, or a little piece of bread?" Or a little piece of "you fill in the blank." If it isn't water, the answer is no! A true fast is NOTHING BUT WATER and more specifically, pure water.

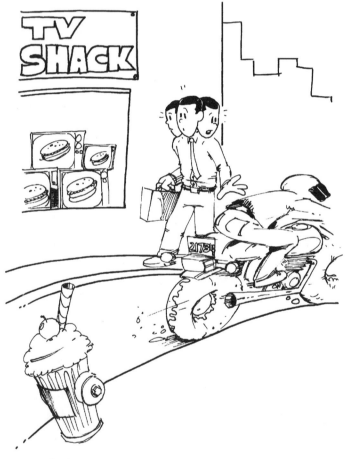

We may talk about sex being the strongest fleshly drive, but it is not. We may think ego is the strongest of the fleshly impulses, but it is not. From the day we are born, the desire for food reigns dominant.

Chapter 2

WHY FAST?

(The Spiritual)

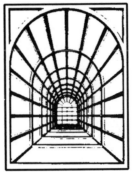

In a spiritual setting the emphasis is often on the denial of the self and the carnal desires to allow us to become more sensitive to God. Food is man's greatest carnal impulse. Many believe that sex is the strongest fleshly drive, but it is not. We may think ego is the strongest of the fleshly impulses, but it is not. From the day we are born, the desire for food reigns dominant.

As newborn infants we first seek the love, comfort and warmth of our mothers, then we cry for food. The sex drive does not develop until the onset of puberty, our teenage years. Sex is the last drive to arrive and the first one to leave. The food drive is present from the beginning to the end, it never leaves, it never disappears. The latest U.S. government study shows that over 60% of all Americans are overweight.

We eat too much. Gluttony, the lack of discipline of the appetite, causes us to look old prematurely, to feel old before we get old and to suffer many different diseases.

All the major killer diseases of today, heart disease, stroke, cancer, diabetes, kidney failure, prematurely kill the majority of Americans and their sources are traceable to our lifestyles and diets. Science has found that it's just as important that we don't overeat, as it is that we eat properly.

Let me repeat that — studies have found that it's as important that we not eat to excess, as it is that we eat properly.

Fasting allows us to gain control of the appetite. When you can develop the discipline to fast, you automatically develop the discipline not to overeat. When you can control your strongest carnal appetite (the desire for food), you can then gain control of the other carnal appetites.

There are many different spiritual reasons why people or groups fast. Sometimes it is to show unity for a cause such as a fast against war, or injustice, or a host of other social ills. Fasting in a group allows you to achieve something that you would never achieve on your own. You can draw on the strength, the determination, the support, and the prayers of the group. Some fast at preset intervals, once per week, once per month, one month per year, etc. Some fast when the social or spiritual need arises. Some fast because the minister said so.

There are many different reasons to fast.

It is important to remember when you fast for spiritual reasons:

FASTING DOES NOT CHANGE GOD!

FASTING CHANGES YOU!

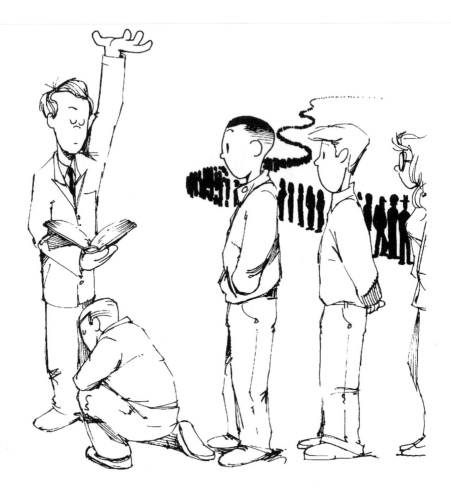

    Americans are sick. Everything from Arthritis to Zits, you name it, we've got it. The church is no exception. Ever been to a church when a well-known healer comes to visit? Have you ever noticed how long the healing line is?

Chapter 3
WHY FAST?
The Physical

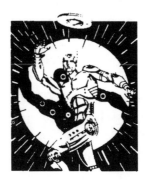

Anything that God ordains has benefits for us here on earth. Yes, fasting has great spiritual benefits but there are very real and tangible rewards in the flesh, or shall I say for our flesh. Fasting, when properly done, can provide great benefits for our physical bodies.

Americans are sick. Everything from Arthritis to Zits, you name it, we've got it. The church is no exception. Ever been to a church when a well-known healer comes to visit? Have you ever noticed how long the healing line is? Come back to that church a year later and look at the line. It will be just as long, with many of the same people in it.

God did not intend for us to be sick. He did not originally intend for us to be healed because we should not have been sick in the first place. You only need healing if you are sick. Man was cast out of the Garden of Eden, cast out of perfect harmony, cast out of a perfect life, and cast out of perfect health when he (or they) ate the wrong thing. We've been eating the wrong things ever since then.

When we eat the wrong things, we eventually get sick, or at least do not have the health and vitality that we should possess. Proper fasting allows God through nature to heal the body. Look at nature for a minute.

If you have a cat or a dog, think about their behavior. If you do not have a cat or dog, then ask someone who does and they will verify what I'm going to tell you. What happens when a cat or a dog gets sick? What do they eat?

Think about this VERY CAREFULLY!

What do they eat when they are sick? Is it PUPPY CHOW®? NINE LIVES®? GRAVY TRAIN®? PUSS 'N BOOTS®? Well, what do they eat? Anyone that has a cat or dog can tell you instantly what they eat when they are sick.

ABSOLUTELY NOTHING!

NO ANIMAL IN NATURE
EATS FOOD WHEN IT IS SICK,
EXCEPT YOU—KNOW—WHO!

Animals instinctively, automatically know what is best for them and they **FAST!** Man is the only creation on the earth that will force himself to eat when he is sick, all of God's other creations know better. They fast.

Man possesses a higher intelligence and is in an entirely different category than the other animals but our bodies work remarkably similar. That is why scientific researchers can test pre-market products on animals. They know the animals' bodies react just as ours do. What hurts their bodies hurts ours and what heals their bodies also heals ours.

I am not advocating animal testing but the connection is undeniable. Their bodies respond similarly to ours.

The same principles of basic health apply. The same foods affect different species of animals with similar metabolic processes and digestive systems in the same way. What causes animals (with similar metabolic processes and digestive systems to ours) to get sick also causes us to get sick. What causes them to get well, causes us to get well. If their bodies work like ours, their bodies will react like ours. You don't need a medical research degree to figure that out.

Fasting is a natural instinct among the animal kingdom when something is wrong with their bodies. They know to stop eating. We may not feel hungry when we are sick but we have been conditioned to eat for strength and to get well.

The digestion of food, especially the typical American diet, takes a tremendous amount of energy. That is why after a big meal you feel sleepy. It can take several days for the typical meal to pass through your body. It takes all of your energy trying to digest that big meal. The body works overtime.

When the body stops digesting food, digestion energy is transferred to do other things. It is those "OTHER THINGS" that the body does with this energy that makes a fast so beneficial.

The minute the digestion energy is released from digestion, the body starts to use it. What does your body do with it? It starts to do primarily ONE THING. It is this one thing that makes fasting so powerful and yet so dangerous. This one thing allows for miraculous cures and instant recoveries of all types of diseases. Once it is understood, there is nothing magical about it. It is simple, but most things of great power are at the root, simple.

This one thing can make such a transformation in your life and health that you will become a permanent believer in the power of fasting for your health.

This one thing, if not understood, can also make you never want to try fasting again. It is nothing new but most people have never heard of it. Most ministers have never spoken on it. Most doctors are even unaware of its mechanism or that it exists. Any fasting book for health will talk about it, but most of us have never read a book on the PHYSICAL HEALTH aspects of fasting.

This is the ONE PRINCIPLE that you must thoroughly understand and know! If you do not understand this, ignorance can discourage, discomfort, or KILL YOU!

Chapter 4

The Most Important Thing To Know About Fasting

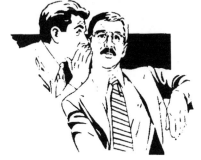

This one thing is the foundational knowledge for fasting for health.

Listen to it!   Digest It!   Remember It!

THIS IS IT!

When you stop eating,

        the body starts to purify itself

                and eliminate toxins!

Upon this law rest all the laws of the healing of the body through fasting.

This law sounds simple, it is. It has profound meaning and effect. It is because of this that the major medical benefit of fasting takes place (besides the spiritual aspects). **When the body stops taking in food, it starts to eliminate the filth and the toxins.**

YOU MUST UNDERSTAND THIS!

It is because of this effect, that I shall call **"FAST FLUSH"**, that we experience many of the so called "bad" effects of a fast. When **FAST FLUSH** starts to occur, we can feel terrible. Can you imagine how much undesirable residue builds up in your body over the years? Years of smoking or breathing in smoke and pollution-filled air carries pollutants to the lungs, then to the bloodstream, then to the tissues.

We have years of eating dead and diseased foods. Our foods are filled with chemical preservatives and additives, chemical perfumes, dyes and such, and all of this is housed in the tissues of our bodies. It is understandable that cancer is on a rampage when it was virtually unheard of 100 years ago.

It is understandable that our skin is drier than ever, needing moisture but unable to get it. Look at the lotion section in your drug or grocery store and see how many of the lotions are now for Extra Dry Skin. As our tissues become laden with chemical overload, we are drying from the inside out.

No one needs to point out the condition of our environment, the quality of our food supply, and the health crisis in the nation. What we need is help in cleansing ourselves of the filth. The FAST FLUSH is one such way. God's infinite intelligence designed a self-cleansing mechanism within us, all we have to do is turn on the self cleaning button. You can not cook in a self-cleaning oven while it is cleaning itself.

This is also true with the human body. You can not continue to stuff food into it while it is trying to purify itself.

Let me explain how the **FAST FLUSH** system works.

In a nutshell, "I don't know." No one else knows either, they just know that it works. When the body "fasts," it "flushes."

We all go through a mini **FAST FLUSH** each night. When we sleep, the body goes into **FAST FLUSH** mode and tries to detoxify itself and get rid of the poisons. When we wake up in the morning we notice it as **"Morning Breath."** It is the **FAST FLUSH** process beginning.

**The more polluted your body,
the more the FAST FLUSH will bring out.**

This principle can not be overemphasized because it is so important and it is the basis of healthful fasting.

**The FAST FLUSH effect
is also the dangerous part.**

When a person fasts, it is not the lack of nutrition or STARVATION that is the danger. The danger is the elimination of toxins that can dump **DECADES** of accumulated poisons in the bloodstream and colon and could literally cause you to die of TOXIC SHOCK.

You will not die of starvation, not in America at least. Let me make clear the difference between fasting and starving, **THEY ARE NOT THE SAME!**

Fasting is the voluntary abstinence from food for a time while the body feeds upon its fat, waste, and stored energy in the form of glycogen. When that fat, waste, and stored energy are used up, then the body will begin to feed upon healthy lean tissue and that's when the body enters into the state called starvation.

Television shows pictures of children from impoverished countries with swollen bellies and bald heads. They are undergoing starvation, which is severe malnutrition.

I spent a week at the beach in Florida while fasting. Guess what I saw strolling up and down the beach day and night. I saw men, executive, well to do men, strolling in bathing suits with swollen bellies and bald heads. A different country, different circumstances, different extremes, but the same effect, **SEVERE MALNUTRITION!** Eating food with NO NUTRITION has similar results as having nothing to eat all.

A person who is fasting is **NOT STARVING.** If they continued until they used up all of their fat, wastes, and energy reserves they would enter into a state of starvation, but that rarely happens and that is not where the danger lies. The body will give signs when it is about to go into starvation. Most people have so much fat on them that they would have to fast over 40 days before their bodies even thought about going into starvation. **The real danger for the average faster is in the poisons that are released, not starvation.**

FAST FLUSH is real.
FAST FLUSH happens
and it will happen to you when you fast.

When we stop eating, all of the energy that is normally directed into digestion is freed. The body then begins the process of trying to eliminate poisonous waste.

We think of the organs of elimination as only being the bowels (colon) and the urinary system. If we do not urinate it out or have a bowel movement (BM) we think that it does not come out. That's not true. There are other organs of elimination. "What others?", I hear you asking. "All I do is urinate and BM."

The largest organ in the body is also an organ of elimination. The skin is the largest organ in the body (yes, the skin is considered an organ) and it is an organ of elimination. The most usual form is perspiration (sweat). When the other organs of elimination can't handle the load or if they are somehow clogged and inefficient, then **Multiple Emissions of Systemic Sanitation or M.E.S.S.** for short, must come out through the skin.

M.E.S.S. causes pimples, zits, acne, blotches, blemishes, pustules, dryness, and a host of other skin problems. The M.E.S.S. comes out through the skin. When M.E.S.S. comes out on the skin, it not only causes the skin to look bad, yes, you guessed it, it causes the skin or the person in the skin to SMELL BAD, too. Now the bad smell is actually caused by the bacteria that grows on the M.E.S.S. once it comes out on the skin, but it all boils down to the same thing. One thing that you will likely notice during a fast is a marked increase in body odor of the offensive smelling kind. The body is trying to purify itself. **DO NOT BE ALARMED.** That is why it is vitally important to understand the main principle of fasting,

When you stop eating, the body starts to purify itself

and eliminate toxins or M.E.S.S.!

The M.E.S.S. does not smell good coming out. You may find that your body odor increases drastically during the first phase of a fast. Mine started after only two days of the pre-fast preparation. Because I understood the **FAST FLUSH** phenomenon it did not concern me. In fact, I felt good about it because I knew this was only my body purifying itself and the odor was only M.E.S.S. poisons being eliminated from my body. I did not try to cover up the odor with deodorant. An antiperspirant would only slow down the process by blocking in the very M.E.S.S. I was trying to get rid of. Just keep your distance from people or at least have them informed of what is happening within your body.

Often the M.E.S.S. toxins coming out through your skin can cause a temporary rash as the body purges them from your system. The M.E.S.S. toxins do not look good coming out either.

The story of the M.E.S.S. toxins coming out gets worse, or better, depending on how you look at it.

Not only can the M.E.S.S. toxins come out through your skin but they also come out through another organ of elimination, the lungs. When a person drinks alcohol or eats garlic, both have one thing in common. Both alcohol and garlic enter the bloodstream.

When they enter the bloodstream, each releases its chemical directly from the bloodstream into the lungs. Then it goes from the lungs straight to your breath. That's why mouthwash and breath mints do not help much with alcohol or garlic.

The chemicals from the alcohol and the garlic are in the bloodstream and it is not a matter of deodorizing, it is a matter of getting them out of the bloodstream.

When the body stops eating, the M.E.S.S. toxins are literally squeezed from the tissues and into the bloodstream.

The bloodstream then struggles to get rid of them any way it can and the first available avenue is often the lungs.

When M.E.S.S. toxins come out through the lungs, simply put. . . your breath will stink. With any fast over three days, I can just about guarantee this will occur. There are ways to minimize the unpleasant body odor social effects of fasting. I will discuss that in the chapter on what to do during the fast.

When FAST FLUSH happens, stuff we never even knew was in our bodies starts to be flushed out. We start to FLUSH out drugs (legal and illegal), nicotine, caffeine, pesticides, preservatives, etc. These chemicals can lie stored in our tissues for longer than we would dare imagine. Many of these toxins have been in our bodies since childhood. None of this M.E.S.S. looks or smells good coming out. It's a blessing that we are getting it out of our bodies before it makes us sick or sicker.

As unpleasant as the body odor and bad breath may sound, that is not the difficult part. "What is worse than that?" I hear you screaming.

How the M.E.S.S. makes you feel
is worse than that.

As the M.E.S.S. toxins impact your bloodstream and flood from your tissues, they can make you feel terrible. You will feel drained, you may be weak, tired, listless, rundown, beat down, and only fit to lie down.

YOU MUST UNDERSTAND WHY!
It is still because of FAST FLUSH.

Your body is going through a massive cleansing. You now have more FREED M.E.S.S. toxins floating in your bloodstream than ever before. Your body is now diverting all available energy to cleansing your system. Yes, you may feel tired. The more toxic your system, the more exhausted you will feel. It is **NOT LACK OF FOOD** that has you weak and exhausted, it is the toxins.

The minute you eat the cleaning process will stop. The M.E.S.S. toxins will stop pouring out. Your breath and body odor will clear up, and things will go back to the toxic condition that you were in before. When this happens people mistakenly believe that "THE FOOD" gave them energy and the fast was draining their energy due to no nourishment. Long term fasters will tell you that the energy usually increases after the 15th day to beyond what it was before the fast began. **ENERGY INCREASES AFTER THEY HAVE GOTTEN THE BULK OF THE M.E.S.S. OUT.**

The temptation to eat due to the effects of M.E.S.S. coming out is great. Eating will eliminate the negative feeling, but enduring to the end of the fast will have a greater positive impact on your health.

Each person's reaction to M.E.S.S. coming out may be different. I tasted metallic chemicals in my mouth for five days during my last fast. I knew what it was. I was tasting chemicals which had been stored in my body for ages. Even though I have never taken any quantity of medicines or drugs in my life, I had untold poisonous pesticide and pollution residues in my tissues. This was because of the environment and contaminated food I had consumed all my life.

If you have a history of heavy pharmaceutical use, the cleansing could be drastic. If your body is extremely toxic, the outpouring M.E.S.S. can cause serious harm. The next chapter deals with simple ways to tell how toxic you are before you begin to fast.

Chapter 5

HOW MUCH OF A TOXIC DUMP ARE YOU?

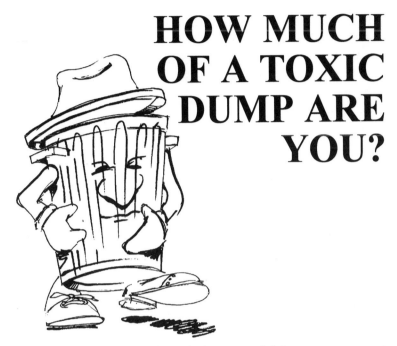

Before attempting to fast, it is a good idea to try to get some idea of exactly how much M.E.S.S. you are carrying around in your system. There are two basic ways to roughly estimate this. Neither is complicated or will involve sophisticated medical equipment. Both are fairly accurate.

When toxins enter the body, the body knows this stuff is not good for it. The body tries to do one of three things with them:

1. Burn them up in metabolic processes (that is, use it for food).
2. Eliminate them through an organ of elimination.
3. Bind them up and store them out of the way for years.

Since the body knows these toxins are not good for it, it recognizes them for what they are: M.E.S.S.

If our bodies can use them for food at least that gets rid

of it. If our bodies can eliminate them, that gets rid of it, too.
If our bodies can't do either of the two, they are left with
only the third option: Put the M.E.S.S. in a form that can be
stored the safest and put them away.

There are two easy methods to determine how much
M.E.S.S. is in you.

For the first method you will need:

1. Full length mirror
2. Privacy
3. Honesty

Get alone in front of the full length mirror. Lock the
door. Take off all of your clothes. Be honest about what you
see.

Look particularly at your midsection. Is it bloated? Is
there a potbelly there? Are there rolls of fat protecting (or
suffocating) your stomach? If there are, then chances are
you are pretty toxic. If your abdominal section is distended,
more than likely it is packed full of dead and decaying material that is highly toxic.

Question:
***Do you have a bowel movement for each meal that
you eat?***

Yes, you should have a bowel movement for each meal
that you eat. Regular is **NOT ONCE A DAY,** regular is
ONCE PER MEAL. Think again about your cat or dog.
They have a bowel movement for each meal that they eat.
So should you.

If the answer to the distended stomach question is yes
and the answer to the bowel movement question is no,
chances are you are very toxic on the inside.

"But everybody else's stomach looks like this, too, and they don't sit on the commode a bit more than I do!" you say.

You have a valid point but everyone else in hell will not make you cool. America's health is not very good. We have sickness on every hand and in almost every body. Because everyone else is unhealthy does not justify your being unhealthy. Another person's sin does not excuse your own.

The second test is simple also. Again you will need no fancy equipment or trained medical personnel. You probably already know the answer to this one without having to experiment.

HOW DO YOU FEEL
WHEN YOU MISS A MEAL OR TWO?

If you get a headache when you miss a meal, then you are extremely toxic. Fast with just water for 24 hours. If you feel sick, get headaches, or if you are dizzy or extremely weak, you are very toxic. It's normal to feel hunger, but not sickness. If you feel sick it means the FAST FLUSH is really pouring M.E.S.S. toxins into your bloodstream at a very high rate.

If your body shows signs of being extremely toxic, you need to go on a pre-fast regimen before going on a full fast. This will be a lot easier and safer on you and your body. Even the pre-fast regimen will not be easy. When M.E.S.S. comes out, it's not pleasant whether you are in a full fast or not.

The highly toxic condition is where fasting can be dangerous. If you do not gradually reduce the toxins in your body, a full fast can be a devastating shock on the system and it may not be able to handle the toxins that pour forth.

Besides the visual inspection and the 24 hour fast, you can ask yourself a few questions that will give you insight as to whether your body may be highly toxic.

A yes answer to these questions means a higher probability of high toxicity and a greater need for a pre-fast regimen.

1. Are you a current or former smoker?
2. Do you work or socialize around smokers?
3. Do you eat much meat?
4. Do you eat many dairy products?
5. Do you have less than one bowel movement per meal?
6. Are you presently on, or have you ever been on, heavy medications or drugs (legal or illegal)?
7. Do you not exercise regularly?
8. Are you more than 20 pounds overweight?
9. Do you drive in congested traffic or live near air pollution?
10. Do you drink less than eight glasses of water daily?
11. Do you eat less than five servings of fresh fruit and fresh vegetables daily?
12. Do you work in an industrial environment with a lot of chemicals?
13. Do you take laxatives?
14. Does your family have a history of short life span?
15. Do you have constant mucus (stuffy nose, sinus congestion, cannot breathe through nostrils clearly, etc.)?
16. Do you have a "bad" body odor without deodorant?
17. Do you have "bad breath" and constantly chew gum to cover it up?
18. Do you get sick easily and have many colds?
19. Do you have a major illness?
20. Do you have many minor illnesses such as arthritis, bad skin (psoriasis, acne, etc.)?

Go through these 20 questions. Many yes answers indicate the probability of a highly toxic body.

Fasting can do wonders in such conditions but the cautions must be observed. The body has to be slowly and safely detoxified.

You must remember, you did not become toxic overnight, it took many years. Do not expect to clean it overnight. If you have been clogging it up for 40 years, at least allow one day per year of your age to clean it out. The next chapter deals with a pre-fast regimen.

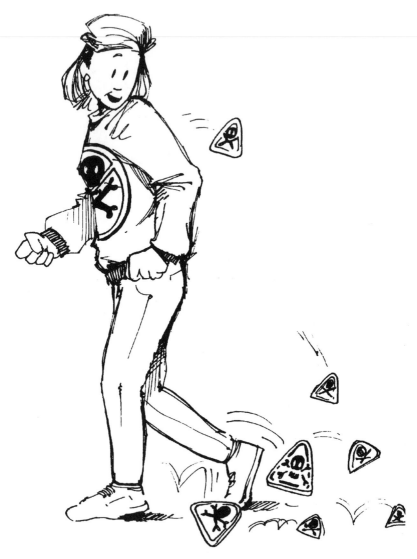

The pre-fast program is strictly to REDUCE the level of toxicity in the body to a point where a full fast will not be harmful.

Chapter 6

THE PRE FAST PROGRAM

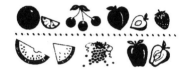

In the previous chapter "HOW MUCH OF A TOXIC DUMP ARE YOU?" we discussed how to determine your level of toxicity. The pre-fast program is strictly to REDUCE the level of toxicity in the body to a point where a full fast will not be harmful. The more toxic your body is, the longer the pre-fast program should be.

The pre-fast program is in itself a fast. Although not a full fast, the pre-fast program performs a milder version of what the full fast does. There are many different types of pre-fast programs. Different health professionals will favor different versions but there is one that is agreed upon by almost everyone. It's taken straight from the Bible. Some would call it a fruit fast. I like to call it "The Eden Diet."

> *And God said, Behold, I have given you every herb bearing seed, which is upon the face of all the earth, and every tree, in the which is the fruit of a tree yielding seed; to you it shall be for meat.*
>
> *Gen. 1:29*

The rule is simply this: If it fits what God allowed in the Garden of Eden when man was in perfection, then eat it.

As I mentioned, I am a Christian, so I am partial to a particular spiritual viewpoint and set of scriptures. No matter what your spiritual beliefs are, the principles are what natural health experts recommend and they work. Fasting is universal in its spiritual or non-spiritual application.

So if it is raw (not cooked, pasteurized, or processed in any way), not of an animal but of herbal (plant) origin, you can eat it. That's it, that's the Eden Diet. That also means NO SALT and NO SUGAR!!!

All questions about what you can eat on The Eden Diet are answerable with, "Sure it's OK to eat, as long as it's an herb (meaning plant) and as long as it's not cooked or altered in any way."

What about vegetables . . . sure it's OK to eat, as long as it's an herb (meaning plant) and as long as it's not cooked or altered in any way.

What about nuts . . . sure it's OK to eat, as long as it's an herb (meaning plant) and as long as it's not cooked or altered in any way. Go easy on the nuts though. Nuts are concentrated protein foods and are rather difficult to digest. In addition, there is not much water in nuts. High water content foods are a necessity since they are the foods that flush the body.

What about fruit juices. . .   isn't that altered from the garden? Yes, but . . . sure it's OK to eat, as long as it's an herb (meaning plant) and as long as it's not cooked or altered in any way. Eat the fruit whole, (you need the fiber) just the way it was intended from the garden.

What about bread. . . that isn't from the garden.

What about honey. . . what plant makes honey?

The Eden Diet is an excellent pre-fast program. It's simple and it works. The enzymes from the fresh unaltered and uncooked fruits and vegetables work wonders on the system. Yes, vegetables can be eaten uncooked and raw.

It's interesting that cooked corn often goes through the digestive system with the kernels still intact. **When corn is eaten raw, it's all digested, there are no kernels left in the stool.** Raw corn is sweet too, where do you think they get corn syrup to sweeten so much stuff from? Okra, broccoli, and other vegetables can all be eaten raw. They flush out the body in many ways and prepare the body for the full fast.

Citrus fruits are especially good for this. Oranges, lemons, limes, grapefruits, and tangerines all work within the body to neutralize the toxins and get them out of the body. The other rule of The Eden Diet: Eat one thing at a time and allow at least 20 to 30 minutes between different types of foods.

The one food at a time is nature's way. Again notice, only man combines more than one type of food at a meal. All animals in nature eat ONE THING at a time. The single food allows for greater and faster detoxifying than eating combination of foods.

You may even notice some of the same effects of the FAST FLUSH with The Eden Diet. The Eden Diet will not only begin the detox process, but if maintained long enough, will cause many miraculous self healings in itself. No doctor can cure you. Doctors do not have the power to heal. Only God can do that and he has placed the power within your own body and within the foods that have been placed in the garden for you.

How long should you continue on
The Eden Diet
before you begin the full fast?

First, you can not overdue The Eden Diet!

You could stay on The Eden Diet for the rest of your life and you would be healthier and live longer than if you ate the Standard American Diet. Compared to **The SAD Diet**, **The Eden Diet** would guarantee you as full a life as possible. If you stay on The Eden Diet your health should be just about perfect and disease free.

So how long do you stay on The Eden Diet? For at least as many days as you intend to fast or until the FAST FLUSH symptoms disappear. When the FAST FLUSH symptoms of bodily cleansing disappear, you know that your body has reached a certain level of cleanliness. The shock of the full fast will be abated tremendously by this initial cleansing with The Eden Diet.

Pre-fast preparation is **VERY IMPORTANT** to minimize the discomfort of a fast. The cleaner your body, the fewer problems you will have. The more toxic your body, the greater the discomfort of the FAST FLUSHING process. **Remember, it is NOT the lack of nourishment that will cause problems during a fast, it is the release of toxins into the system**.

Please note the warning on page four for diabetics as well as those with ulcers. These are special conditions that make it inadvisable to fast. Any person with serious illness should ALWAYS consult a physician or, even better, a natural practitioner with fasting knowledge and experience before attempting a fast. That brings us to the next chapter.

Chapter 7

Consulting A Doctor

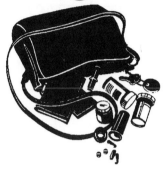

All books on the subject of fasting that I have read advise you to consult a doctor before beginning a fast, especially if you are sick.

Most fasters for non-religious reasons are persuaded towards natural living, natural foods, natural environments, and natural medicines. Generally those that lean towards the natural, move away from orthodox or standard medicine.

They often do not trust the money driven, drug and surgery dependent medical establishment. Why then do they all say consult your doctor first before going on a fast? There is a simple answer to that.

I would be willing to say that most medical doctors have:
1. Never been on a fast personally.
2. No real belief in fasting for the healing and purifying benefits of a fast.
3. Never truly studied fasting as opposed to starvation and malnutrition.

The usual medical view in the cases of illness is to make the patient eat. If the patient is too weak or too incapacitated to eat, they will put a tube in their veins or directly into their stomach and force feed them. Even if you are in the intensive care coronary unit recovering from a massive heart attack, not only will they bring you lots of food, but lots of greasy food. If you have visited people in the hospital then you know that this is true. Modern medicine does not provide you with a healthy diet in what is *supposed* to be the epitome of healing places, the hospital. Even the word "hospital" itself comes from the root word "hospice", which means "a place to die".

Doctors are necessary in this society. Most are honest, dedicated, hard working people. Maybe modern medicine has not moved in the direction of natural cures because that's not what the patient wants.

If we are stricken by the most common of the killers of Americans, the heart attack, we want drugs. We want a shot, or a pill that will make the problem, or at least the pain, go away, and go away without sacrifice or effort on our part.

> **We do not want to hear the doctor say:**
> **Stop smoking**
> **Stop eating fried foods**
> **Stop eating fatty foods**
> **Stop eating salt**
> **Stop drinking alcohol**
> **Stop eating so much that you remain fat**
> **Start exercising regularly**
> **Start eating low calorie healthy foods**
> **Get lean get fit get sweaty,**
> **Throw away the TV remote control**
> **Walk in the fresh air**
> **Push away from the table and live**

The public does not want to hear these words at all. The public wants to eat, drink, and be merry, then die.

A reporter attended a convention of cardiologists (heart specialists). The reporter decided to follow some cardiologists to see how they ate. She was shocked at how many of the cardiologists ate the greasy hamburgers and fries at the local "fast food" hamburger outlet at the convention center. It was against everything that these specialist taught about how to eat! When the reporter interviewed several cardiologists about their dietary habits they said in essence, "It's easy to tell someone else how to eat, it's a lot harder to do it yourself."

Doctors are not required to take nutrition courses. They are not required to know a thing about fasting. They may or may not know about fasting, and the answer is more likely "they don't know". Why then do all of the natural healing oriented promoters of fasting always tell you to check with your doctor before you fast?

FOR THE EXACT SAME REASON I WILL TELL YOU TO CHECK WITH YOUR DOCTOR BEFORE YOUR FAST!

Because if something bad happens to you on the fast, you cannot say I didn't tell you to check with your doctor.

It's a precaution that does have its merits. Unsupervised fasting can be dangerous. Modern medicine can be more dangerous. Just as fasting experts tell you to consult your doctor to determine risks, ask your doctor to let you see the **"contraindications"** on the medicines they give you.

The contraindications are a <u>VERY LONG</u> list of things that can go wrong when you take a medicine. Every medicine that a doctor will give you has them. The contraindicators can be anything from a rash or headache, to death.

The list is usually quite long with all medicines. We call contraindications simply "SIDE EFFECTS." This is the stuff that can happen that we do not want to happen. The list of side effects are "POSSIBLE" side effects. Some side effects are rare, some are common. Some are very mild and just a mere nuisance, some can put you in the ground. Medicines can be VERY dangerous. There is risk in all cures. Especially the farther one moves away from what is naturally in the earth.

To illustrate what I mean, drugs and their side effects are listed below from <u>THE PILL BOOK</u> and The U.S. Pharmacopoeia. According to surveys of chain drug stores, mail order, and drug wholesalers, these are the 10 most prescribed drugs in America.

Each of the medicines are listed with their most common classification or use followed by the side effects. This does not include the other warnings that describe under which conditions not to take the medicine and what other drugs not to mix them with.

Remember these are the top selling drugs at the moment, this means these are most likely among the SAFEST of the drugs.

Along with its needed effects, a medicine may cause some unwanted effects. Although not all of these side effects may occur, if any do occur you may need medical attention.

Remember, these are the side effects that the drug companies **tell you** about!
1. **Amoxil** (penicillin-type drug) - stomach upset, nausea, vomiting, diarrhea, rash, hairy tongue, itching or irritation around the anus and/or vagina.

2. Lanoxin (for heart disease) - loss of appetite, nausea, vomiting, diarrhea, blurred or disturbed vision, and enlargement of the breasts.

3. Xanax (tranquilizer) - aggravates narrow angle glaucoma, mild drowsiness, confusion, depression, lethargy, disorientation, headache, inactivity, slurred speech, stupor, dizziness, tremor, constipation, dry mouth, nausea, inability to control urination, sexual difficulties, irregular menstrual cycle, changes in heart rhythm, lowered blood pressure, fluid retention, blurred or double vision, itching, rash, hiccups, nervousness, inability to fall asleep, and liver dysfunction.

4. Zantac (anti-ulcer drug) - headache, dizziness, constipation, abdominal discomfort, rash, feeling of ill health, reduction in white blood cells or blood platelets, and could cause hepatitis.

5. Premarin (estrogen) - increased risk of certain types of cancer, may increase tendency for blood clots, liver cancer and other liver tumors, high blood pressure, glucose intolerance or development of a symptom similar to diabetes, or the aggravation of diabetes. Breakthrough bleeding, spotting, changes in menstrual flow, dysmenorrhea, premenstrual-type syndrome, amenorrhea, swelling of the ankles and legs, vaginal infection with candida, cystitis-like syndrome, enlargement or tenderness of the breasts, nausea, vomiting, abdominal cramps, feeling of bloatedness, jaundice or yellowing of the skin or whites of the eyes, rash, loss of scalp hair, development of new hairy areas, lesions of the eye, intolerance to contact lenses, headache (possibly migraine), dizziness, depression, weight changes, retention of water, changes in sex drive, stroke, blood clot formation, dribbling or sudden passage of urine, loss of coordination, chest pains, leg pains, difficulty breathing, slurred speech, vision changes, skin rash, skin irritation and redness.

6. **Dyazide** (diuretic-prescribed for high blood pressure or any condition where it is desirable to eliminate water from the body) - Loss of appetite, drowsiness, lethargy, headache, gastrointestinal upset, cramping and diarrhea, rash, mental confusion, fever, feeling of ill health, inability to achieve or maintain erection in males, bright red tongue, burning inflamed feeling in the tongue, headache, tingling in the toes and fingers, restlessness, anemias or other effects on components of the blood, unusual sensitivity to sunlight, dizziness when rising quickly from a sitting position, muscle spasms, gout, weakness, and blurred vision.

7. **Tagamet** (anti-ulcer) - mild diarrhea, muscle pains and cramps, dizziness, skin rash, nausea and vomiting, headache, confusion and drowsiness, impotence (men), and painful swollen breasts. Effects of white blood cells or blood platelets include unusual bleeding or bruising, unusual tiredness or weakness.

8. **Tenormin** (high blood pressure and angina) - dizziness, tingling of the scalp, nausea, vomiting, upset stomach, taste distortion, fatigue, sweating, male impotence, urinary difficulty, bronchial spasms, muscle weakness, cramps, dry eyes, blurred vision, skin rash, hair loss, facial swelling, mental depression, disorientation, short-term memory loss, emotional instability, aggravation of lupus erythematosus, stuffy nose, chest pains, colitis, drug allergy, (fever, sore throat), and unusual bleeding or bruising.

9. **Naprosyn** (relief of pain and inflammation) - stomach upset, dizziness, headache, drowsiness, ringing in the ears, heartburn, nausea, vomiting, bloating, gas in the stomach,

stomach pain, diarrhea, constipation, dark stool, nervousness, insomnia, depression, confusion, tremor, loss of appetite, fatigue, itching, rash, double vision, abnormal heart rhythm, anemia or other changes in the composition of the blood, changes in liver function, loss of hair, tingling in the hands and feet, fever, breast enlargement, lowered blood sugar, and effects on the kidneys.

10. Cardizem (angina, high blood pressure, prevention of reoccurrence of some kinds of heart attack) - abnormal heart rhythms, fluid accumulation in the hands, legs, or feet, headache, fatigue, nausea, rash, low blood pressure, dizziness, fainting, changes in heart rate, heart failure, light-headedness, nervousness, tingling in the hands or feet, hallucinations, temporary memory loss, difficulty sleeping, weakness, diarrhea, vomiting, constipation, upset stomach, itching, unusual sensitivity to sunlight, painful or stiff joints, liver inflammation, and increased urination.

These are the top 10 prescription drugs from *THE PILL BOOK*. *(drug names are trademarks of their respective manufacturers)* Anyone that takes prescription medication should have a copy of this book. It gives detail descriptions of the 1,600 most commonly prescribed drugs in the United States. If you are going to take these drugs, you should know the possible side effects.

All of these top 10 warn "do not take this drug if you have had an allergic reaction to it." Of course, the only way to know if you are allergic to the drug is if you have already had a bad reaction to it or something similar to it. Too often, that one bad reaction is enough and too much. That one bad allergic reaction can KILL you. There is another warning on the top 10 that's also scary.

ALL OF THE TOP TEN DRUGS
PASS THROUGH IN BREAST MILK!

Many of them pass through in the blood stream but ALL of them pass through in breast milk. The same reactions that an adult can have, so can an infant if the mother breast fed the child or was pregnant with the child while taking the prescription.

The same can also be said of general toxins or M.E.S.S. in a woman's body, it passes through to the child. That's just another reason why a woman would want her bloodstream and body detoxified and FAST FLUSHED, to provide a clean environment for her child.

I have listed these top 10 to show you that even though fasting can have side effects, SO CAN ANYTHING YOU GET FROM A DOCTOR!

There is still no true count of the deaths caused by prescription drug reactions. Considering the alternatives, if done in time, fasting is a safer method of cleansing the body and getting on the road to being disease free than any medicine from a prescription pad.

Go see a doctor, but ask your doctor at least two questions.

1. Have you ever fasted?
2. Do you really know anything about fasting?

If they answer no to both questions then go see another doctor. You will probably have to visit a doctor that specializes in natural medicine and natural healing methods. Look in the yellow pages, but find a specialist that knows what they are doing concerning fasting.

I honestly would recommend that anyone, (especially with a very toxic body), see a doctor **(a doctor that really KNOWS about fasting, not just ANY doctor)** before beginning a LONG fast. Short fasts (under five days) should not be a health danger for the vast majority, **ESPECIALLY IF THEY FOLLOW THE INSTRUCTIONS IN THIS BOOK!**

It's amazing that of the many destructive things that we do to our bodies, we never consulted a doctor before starting them. Equally amazing, they are against all Biblical and other religious teaching.

Did you ask a doctor before you . . .

◆ smoked - cigarettes, crack, or marijuana?
◆ had unprotected sex with someone you weren't absolutely sure didn't have a disease?
◆ ate that greasy heart clogging digestive system cluttering meal?
◆ drove that car with no seat belt?
◆ had those six-packs and got drunk?
◆ let that potbelly budge out in front?

No, you didn't, did you?

God did not ordain or condone ANY of those behaviors but you did not ask a doctor before you did them. Yet everyone tells you to ask a doctor before you fast. What God ordained, they want you to ask a doctor about.

God ordained fasting. Jesus said *"when ye fast"* NOT "IF," BUT *"WHEN YE FAST"* Matthew 6:16. The instruction and correctness of fasting did not come from natural healing doctors or ancient medicine. They recognized the benefits and the correctness of fasting, but they didn't originate it.

Fasting came out of the spiritual tradition of ALL the major religions. Whether you are one of the sixty something different denominations of Christianity, or Islamic, Hindu or Buddhist, fasting is strongly suggested in all major religions and commanded in some.

It was not man's invention. It came from a higher surgeon general. Then why do we need to ask a doctor if we should do something God ordained for us to do?

If I had to have side effects, I would rather get them from something God instructed me to do than from the needle or pill of man's medicine. Fasting's side effects are the results of purification. The side effects of drugs are the result of increasing the toxicity already in the body.

Read the list (the list the doctors are given by the drug companies) of the side effects of the top drugs again. The list may change every decade, but the side effects remain essentially the same. That same list of side effects will be just as accurate 100 years from now, only the top ten drugs will change.

Ask a doctor, but ask a doctor that knows about fasting, better still, ask a doctor that has personal experience with fasting. For even though I had read much about fasting, I did not believe much of what I read until I experienced it.

You will find that the greatest doctor of all has already been given to you.

Chapter 8

THE FAST

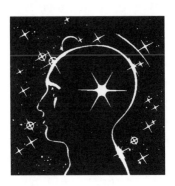

If this is your first fast, I would recommend a very short fast to start with, especially if you rate high on the toxic list.

Even if you did not rate high on the toxic list, it is generally **NOT A GOOD IDEA TO START ANY POTENTIALLY DIFFICULT UNDERTAKING AT AN EXTREME.** If you decided to start jogging, you would not go out and run a 26.2 mile marathon as your first exercise would you?

You would start by running around the block. Then you would run one mile, then two, then three, until you gradually increased your endurance to the level that you desired. So it is with fasting.

You should not start with a 40 day fast. You may never want to attempt a 40 day fast, just as most joggers never attempt to run a 26 mile marathon. Most joggers run a few miles. That is sufficient to keep them in the physical condition that they desire. They do not wish to be in marathon condition.

You may have no desire (or need) for an extended fast. Fasting is a personal experience done for many different reasons. There is no reason why a healthy person could not jump straight into a long fast, if it is conducted correctly. Many of the health clinics that specialize in fasting cures would routinely put patients that had never fasted before on a 21 day water fast.

Remember, however, that those patients were monitored constantly by a professional. They were also usually secluded in a very peaceful and restful environment with an abundance of emotional support. It can be done without a doubt, but I do not recommend it.

Most who attempted a long fast (over 7 to 14 days) fail. The reason is not that they physically could not make it, but they psychologically fail.

Just as geese in formation can fly 75 percent farther than they can alone, the average person can fast better with someone else for support than they can alone.

Those in the Christian faith may say that Jesus was alone when he fasted for 40 days and nights in the wilderness. Well, he was not exactly alone, the devil was with him. *(Luke 4:2).* When you fast, temptation will walk side by side with you also.

Moses was alone when he fasted twice on the mountain for 40 days and 40 nights with neither food nor water.

No! You can not fast without drinking water. Moses was in a mist or cloud in the presence of God. The mist watered Moses *(Exodus 21:18).* If you sat in a bathtub full of water, the water would saturate your skin. It may become wrinkled from water saturation or hydration. So it was with Moses in the midst of a mist.

Elijah was alone when he fasted for 40 days and nights during his journey through the desert *(1 Kings 19:8).*

However, most of us do not have the spiritual strength of the leaders of the Christian faith nor would any other followers of other faiths generally have the spiritual strength of the leaders of those faiths.

To fast alone is best from a spiritual view. During my longest fast, I went away alone. I left my wife and family. I explained that I needed to do as my spiritual leaders had done and go into the wilderness and to the mountains (to nature) and get away. They understood and gave me their blessings.

For the first half of my fast, I went to the ocean and for the second half I went to the mountains. Being alone allows you to reflect, pray, meditate, and deal with things within yourself that you can't accomplish in the constant company of others.

From a practical view it is more difficult to do anything alone versus having someone with you that is on the same accord. If you are new to fasting, it is always easier to have a partner to start with. As you become more experienced, the need for company will decrease.

When I mention partner, I always interject "on the same accord." It is critical that if you are going to tell people that you are going on a fast, they should be people that understand fasting.

Most Americans cringe at the thought of missing more than one day of eating. Many even cringe at not getting three full meals a day (not including snacks at night). Our entire society in inundated with messages of eating, eating and eating.

Watch television for an hour any day of the week. Notice how many commercials are devoted to food. If you tell someone that you will be fasting and they do not understand fasting, you are asking for trouble. They instantly assume that you will drop dead in a few days from starvation. Even if you are 50 pounds overweight, they will think that you will drop dead in a few days from starvation.

Most Americans know very little, if anything, about fasting. They view it as starvation and there are no positive benefits of starvation.

BE VERY CAREFUL
WHO YOU TELL ABOUT YOUR FAST
THEY MIGHT NOT UNDERSTAND

If you fast with someone that is of the same understanding as you about fasting, both of you will strengthen the other. When one gets weak and wants to give up, the other encourages and vice a versa.

Jesus says in Matthew 6:17-18 NIV translation *"But when you fast, put oil on your head and wash your face, so that it will not be obvious to men that you are fasting, but only to your Father, who is unseen; and your Father, who sees what is done in secret, will reward you."*

In this verse the Bible tells you many things about fasting. Some of those require deeper understanding but they coincide very well with what fasting experts say.

As I mentioned in the beginning, you may not be Christian, you may not be of any religion. The purpose of QUICK FASTING is not to preach to you about religion, but to educate you about how to fast. The Bible is the spiritual document that I believe in and know best. The references in other spiritual works do not contradict what the Bible says about fasting. It is not a coincidence that Ramadan (a mandatory fast each year for Islamics) is 40 days. The only specific number of days of fasts mentioned in the Bible is one day, seven days and 40 days.

I use a Christian scriptural reference because that is what I am. An Islamic would use references from the Quran and quotes from Mohammed. A Buddhist would use references from the words of Buddha, etc. Someone of no particular religion may simply rely on health data and results attained from others who have fasted. Fasting works, whether you are an American Indian or from Zaire. Fasting works whether you are A.M.E., Baptist, C.O.G.I.C., or follow Zend-Avesta. Just as eating has certain benefits (or detriments depending on what you eat) that are independent of your religious beliefs, so does fasting.

Now that I've said that, maybe you will not be up in arms if I use a Biblical quote. Back to Matthew 6:17-18 *"But when you fast, put oil on your head and wash your face, so that it will not be obvious to men that you are fasting, but only to your Father, who is unseen; and your Father, who sees what is done in secret, will reward you."*

There are several points here that correlate with what fasting experts tell you to do. You may have to stretch your mind and understanding to get the full impact and meaning of what is being said.

THE OIL

"Put oil on your head" or as The King James Version puts it, *"But thou, when thou fastest, anoint thine head."*

Jesus said to put oil on your head. This has a spiritual significance but I will discuss only the things that universally relate to fasting. Putting oil on during a fast has physical significance as well.

As I was preparing to fast for 40 days, I attended a function where perhaps one of the most famous of the modern day health gurus and, perhaps, the most recognized fasting expert appeared—Dick Gregory.

I was blessed to have a chance after the function for a long discussion with Dick Gregory. Gregory has one of the top selling diet formulas in health food stores (Dick Gregory's Bahamian Diet®). He also has some of the most amazing fasting stories that you will ever hear that include feats of endurance and walking hundreds of miles with NO FOOD. Many have read of his fasting exploits but it is still hard to believe.

Gregory was the one who gave me much of the insight about "asking a doctor." When people asked him if he consulted his doctor before the many fasts of his life, he replied, "Heck no." "My doctor has long been dead."

For most Americans, 40 days without food is almost impossible to believe. I was startled at some of the things he told me. Frankly I had a difficulty believing some of them, particularly concerning MY body. I began to research many of the things he shared, and found written references that verified virtually all he had elaborated upon.

One of the first things he told me was, *"Get yourself some oil because a long fast will cause your skin to dry out."*

Permit me, if you will, a digression here. I need to explain a little about myself and the way I think, my background and what qualifies me to tell you about fasting. There was no resume, or brief summary of the author at the beginning of QUICK FASTING. I think it is important for you to understand how I think. When you understand that, you can then understand my thinking process when Dick Gregory told me to get some oil.

Chapter 9

THIS IS ME
(or at least a certain part)

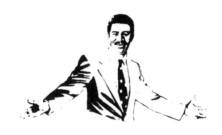

I am a scientist. In 1977, I graduated from Eckerd
College (formerly Florida Presbyterian College) in
St. Petersburg, Florida with a B.S. in Chemistry. I am not
just a scientist by educational training, but one by nature.
There is a difference in a scientist and a technician. A technician takes known procedures and knowledge and routinely
applies them to particular circumstances. Technicians exist
in all walks of life, not just science.

A scientist seeks not to routinely use established knowledge but to find the unknown. They seek to discover the hid-
den, to learn what the masses are ignorant of, and to shed
light where darkness abides. A scientist has a mentality of
seeking, a technician has a mentality of using. Both mental-
ities are necessary and present in every individual but in different proportions.

Knowledge is not limited to science. Knowledge is science. I learned in school the "so called" hierarchy of knowledge. It is an inverted pyramid as follows:

The Knowledge Pyramid
"from my college's point of view"

PHILOSOPHY AND RELIGION
God, Spiritual and the Supernatural
SOCIOLOGY
Groups of bio-systems
PSYCHOLOGY
Mind-Soul with bio-sys
MEDICINE
Malfunction of bio-sys
BIOLOGY
Math, Physics, & Chemistry with Life Force added
CHEMISTRY
Math & Physics applied with Molecular interaction
PHYSICS
Math applied to objects, Relativity involved
MATH
The simplest knowledge. No need for experience

For the *THOROUGH* and *COMPLETE* understanding of each level you *MUST* understand the level below it. If you do not understand the level below it, that does not mean you cannot function at that level. It just means that you do not have complete understanding.

Here's an example of how the hierarchy of knowledge works. Let's look at something we do daily - driving a car.

The Hierarchy of Knowledge of the Basic Automobile

Transmission
(Pressure plate clutch or hydraulically operated automatic with torque converter)
Four cycle internal combustion engine
(the four cycles - intake, compression, explosion, exhaust) (carburetor or fuel injection)
Metallurgy
Ignition and combustion of alkanes
Petroleum (crude oil and it's refinement into gasoline)

Those are just very broad generalizations to get power to the wheels. Do you know exactly where tires come from and how they are made? How metals are smelted and cast? How wire is made? What about the glass for the windshield? What makes the mirror reflective? What makes the turn signals blink? How does the radio tune to each station and how does the amplifier in it work? Each component in itself is a blend of sub-components that is an engineering feat.

Usually, we understand the component as it is and how it BASICALLY functions, not how it came to be or its intricate workings. Our understanding the component as it is dwindles when we try to explain the complete function of it.

Think of the simplest item in a car. Look around your car and find the simplest item. What is it, maybe a knob? That's simple enough isn't it? Well, not exactly. What is it made of? Plastic? What kind of plastic and how is it made? "Uh . . . maybe poly . . . let me see what else is simple." **Maybe there isn't anything really simple. Understand this.**

Creating an automobile involves thousands of processes that the average person or even mechanic has no idea of how they came to be, or what they are. Yet, if every adult were asked if they understood what an automobile was, they would answer, "Of course I know what a car is!"

Almost every adult can drive. They can successfully operate and (some) even repair a car. But our knowledge of things we use every day is very limited when it comes to **THOROUGH** and **COMPLETE** understanding.

QUICK FASTING has nothing to do with cars. It does have something to do with a more thorough and complete understanding. Cars are simple. The knowledge is there for any person that chooses to learn. It is complete, and it is flawlessly reproducible. Cars fit into the first three levels of knowledge. They involve nothing more than math, physics and chemistry and rudimentary biology since many of the raw materials and fuels have organic origins.

This book deals with the top levels. The human body, mind, and spirit makes a car look like a child's set of building blocks. It is similar to the automobile, just infinitely more complicated. I am like a little child riding in a car that I do not completely understand. I hear noises, look out the window, make correlations between what I believe is cause and effect, but I make no claim to thoroughly understand the vehicle. It is not simple.

We may think modern man understands biology and medicine, but do we really? The best doctors and researchers still do not know exactly what causes our leading diseases. Theories abound but we do not know exactly what causes cancer. We still have no cure in sight. We do not know why some get sick and others do not under virtually identical circumstances.

In the ancient days when man did not understand something, he attributed it to the gods. That's why there was a god for every natural occurrence; a rain god, a fertility god, a sun god, a moon goddess, etc., until the nature of the scientist in a few men banished those gods and replaced them with knowledge. Science did not banish the things man does not know, it actually increased our awareness of them. The list is not only long, we don't even know the full list.

I consider myself to be an extremely well-educated and enlightened person. I can safely say that I know more than most. I can also say that I am more aware of my ignorance.

I have given this prelude so you understand that I am about to take you for a ride in a car that I do not **THOROUGHLY** and **COMPLETELY** understand. I don't feel bad about that because neither does anyone else in the flesh thoroughly and completely understand it either. Not doctors, not researchers, not the natural health practitioners, not the government, and no, not even preachers (of which I just happen to be one) COMPLETELY understand anything.

"For we know in part, and we prophesy in part. But when that which is perfect is come, then that which is in part shall be done away." (1 Cor. 13:9-10)

I am not the driver on your fasting trip. I am a passenger with only a certain amount of control over the car. I can help you influence its direction and speed. The road may be very curved. There are twists and turns that can boggle the mind. It is difficult to tell how each journey will end or what territories each traveler will wind through. It will make sense in the end, but getting to the end is not easy. **Buckle your seat belt and unbuckle your mind, this ain't no ordinary ride.**

I don't know what you will think about the truth of fasting. It is true no matter what you think about it. More accurately I should say it is truth from my perspective, knowledge and experience. When I finished my first fast over seven days, my skin was as smooth as a baby's. Family and friends noticed the tremendous change. I know beyond a shadow of a doubt fasting works. That is my story. There are always three sides to every story. The two sides and the truth. This is my side.

What do I do for a living, other than writing? I am a chemist, a pastor, (The ARK of Salvation, hear my sermons at www.theonlineword.com). My main area of expertise is in cosmetic chemistry. I have developed over 70 cosmetic products, many of which are on your grocery and drug store shelves now. I have also created or developed several other products in many different areas.

I have written an electronics book, built a recording studio and produced and engineered four albums, developed an electronic home product, developed a pet product, two computer programs and created a relaxation tape called "SLEEP OF THE WOMB," a relaxation tape and CD that features the actual sounds from the inside of a woman's womb against a background of the sounds of nature. The sounds of the womb causes an infant to sleep, it also relaxes an adult. Yes, it really works!

My company developed several products that you will find in thousands of health food stores. MIRACLE 2000® is what many consider the most amazing nutritional product on the market. Of course I would say that but look at what's in it. The 26 major vitamins and minerals, many at 2000% RDA, 18 herbs, over 70 ionic trace minerals, blue green algae, antioxidants, amino acids, aloe and other nutrients are contained in an easily assimilated and swallowed liquid form. MIRACLE 2000® and LIFESEED® are great tasting liquids, one ounce gives you supplementation that normally requires several products. They are in health food stores.

COLD WAR® is a capsule that provides the body's

immune system with fortification when you need more than chicken soup to fight a cold. MIRACLE OIL® and MIRACLE LOTION® are products that I developed as a natural treatment especially for dry skin. I will talk about these two later as they relate particularly to fasting. HEART MIRACLE™ can be seen online at www.heartmiracle.com.

As you can see, I have quite a varied professional life. I have always made it a point to try to understand things from the ground up.

The more you understand, the more you can do. How did I get from chemistry to a book on fasting? As I said, I am a scientist, a seeker of truth. When you start a journey seeking truth, there are at least two places your journey will take you.

First, where you didn't expect to go.

Second, to a place that won't be crowded when you get there.

Truth began for me with the physical body. At age 17, (I was born on December 31, 1955, so you can figure out how old or young I am now) my father took me to the Natural Hygiene Convention in Rockford, Illinois. We stayed on a college campus for a week. We were taught and lectured by doctors each day. They explained how and why we should live a healthy lifestyle.

The subjects included diet, (why meat, dairy and most processed foods were not in the best interest of your health), exercise, fresh air, peace of mind and of course, fasting.

There was no spirituality involved. It was strict science. We were dealing with medical professionals that were convinced that a natural lifestyle was your best insurance against disease and a premature death.

That one week forever changed my life. Even at 17,

I was a scientist. I could see and understand the statistics. I understood the physiology of the digestive system. The science of proper food combining and the interaction of the digestive juices on different food combinations made sense.

Of the major destructive behaviors, most people know they are destructive. Everyone now knows cigarettes are destructive. We know that excess weight is destructive. We know it is destructive not to exercise regularly. We know living in a smog filled city is destructive. We know fried, fatty foods are destructive. We know refined sugar sweets are destructive. We know violent movies and television shows ultimately are destructive. We know marijuana, crack, cocaine, heroin, etc. are all destructive.

First, the knowledge of good and evil must be attained. When you know something is destructive or harmful, you have attained the knowledge of good and evil.

Second, the knowledge must be acted upon. To know smoking kills you prematurely does you no good if you continue to smoke. To know fatty foods are bad for you does you no good unless you reduce your consumption of them.

The Natural Hygiene Society Convention gave me the knowledge of good and evil when it came to taking care of the body. I became very sensitive to this. I decided at the age of 17, I would use that knowledge of good and evil as it related to health, because quite frankly, I like my body.

It functions and serves me well. When it hurts or is sluggish, I don't like it. Furthermore, it's the only body I have, I cannot trade it in and getting the body fixed is usually painful and expensive. In addition, replacement parts are never as good as the original equipment. I made it a point to take excellent care of my body. I simply decided that I would take better care of my body than I would my car.

Unlike my body, I can always buy or lease another car.

Although I believe in divine miraculous healings, too many people are sick in the church. I believe that a divine healing is only second best. Not getting sick is best of all. Therefore, I concentrated on reading, learning, attending seminars and practicing things to keep my body healthy. Ironically, most Americans are far more concerned about their car's health than they are about their health. Dick Gregory said, "If a news report came out that smoking in your car would corrode your engine, people would stop smoking in their cars. If a report came out that buckling your seat belt would give you two more miles per gallon, people would buckle their seat belts. If the news reported that a local gas station was selling cheap watered gas that would rust your engine, people would avoid that gas station."

Unfortunately, this is true, all too true. We would stop behavior that would endanger our cars, but we will not stop behavior that will endanger our bodies. I care and focus on preserving my body more than I focus on preserving my car. After all, when I finish with my car, I will sell it back to the dealer, and he will sell it to someone, maybe you.

It has been over 20 years since I first attended The Natural Hygiene Convention. In all that time, in all of my research, with all the lectures, not one jot or tidbit of what was taught at the first convention was invalidated. The Natural Hygiene Society was based upon a natural way of living that will never be invalidated or improved upon.

Breastfeeding a baby will never be improved upon. We may get more convenience, fancier and more colorful packaging, freedom to move about in public, fancy advertising and promises of what wonders the new man-made milk that can last on the shelf for years will do. MADison Avenue will promise us anything, make us want anything, then deliver us anything. Unfortunately, the thing it delivers does not really do what we think, nor is it best for us.

The MAD in MADison Avenue may indicate that you've got to be crazy to believe everything that advertising tells you. Man's version of New and Improved may be new, but is usually not improved. No matter how man fiddles with the first food from our birth, the nipple is still best, and there is nothing that we can, or should, do about it.

Much of the knowledge of The Natural Hygiene Society is summed up in what I consider to be the best book on diet and health available, FIT FOR LIFE by Harvey and Marilyn Diamond. FIT FOR LIFE is available in most bookstores.

The Diamonds took the principles of The Natural Hygiene Society and condensed them into an easy to understand format. The Diamonds credit Herbert Shelton, founder of The Natural Hygiene Society, for much of the knowledge that they have. So do I. Much of what I know about fasting, I learned from attending The Natural Hygiene Society Convention Seminars across the country and internationally.

This is a little of my background. I say a little because no person is really known by their business or professional pursuits. The real person is something far more subtle than "what do you do for a living." I am probably quite different from the average chemist since I avoid what are commonly considered chemicals in my own life.

I found fasting while seeking to maintain my vehicle, the one that carries my spirit, not the automobile.

I question things. That leads you to learn, but it can also get you in trouble, especially when people don't want you to know the real answer, the truth.

QUICK FASTING is not about me, but you may need to know something about how I got on this road. You needed to know why I had questions when Dick Gregory told me that my skin would dry out.

Chapter 10

BACK TO THE OIL

"Get yourself some oil because a long fast will cause your skin to dry out," Dick Gregory said.

I perused my mind for any information that would verify that statement. I couldn't think of any. I knew a lot about dry skin and the etiology (causes) of it. I knew a lot because I had spent a considerable amount of time developing a natural product for dry skin.

I knew that dry skin was a disease. It's epidemic now. Although it is not considered serious, dry skin does indicate a problem. Your skin should not be dry. Ideally, you should not need a lotion or oil of any kind. Unfortunately, our bodies are not in an ideal condition.

Dry, scaly, patchy, cracking, peeling, blistering, rough, hard, and itchy skin is not healthy skin. I knew this from common sense as well as my research. Therefore, I will not throw a lot of technical mumbo jumbo at you. I trust the obvious and simple things more. Technical terms like epidermis, dermis and subcutaneous tissue, the various layers of skin, do not really matter.

Skin is dry for one simple reason. It is dry for the same reason anything else is dry. It is dry because it lacks water or moisture. This may sound like an over simplistic explanation, but it is quite accurate. That is what causes dryness, lack of water.

The reason there is a lack of water is where things get more complicated. The major cause of constipation is also a lack of water. If you are constipated, try drinking a gallon of water a day for three days. At the end of those three days, you won't be constipated. When things get dry they also get hard (well, not all things). Dryness causes things to get pasty and stiff. You would be surprised at how many things would be cured by simply drinking a sufficient amount of water each day.

During a fast, you must drink a lot of water. I knew Dick Gregory knew that I would do this, so why did he say my skin would dry out? This I could not understand. I thought he had either made a mistake or thought that I would fast without drinking much water. My skin dry out? No way!

Guess what? It dried out.

After the seventh day of fasting, my skin was noticeably dry. Why? I am not sure nor have I been able to find anyone else who knows. I have a theory, but it is only a theory. I know that the toxic M.E.S.S. coming out can cause rashes and bumps. I have personally experienced that.

It stands to reason that if a toxic body can cause dry skin without fasting (and it does, just look at the dry skin lotions on the store shelves) then toxins coming out may cause dry skin, too. Toxins cause the skin to dry for two reasons:

First reason :
The body always channels resources to the body parts that are the most critical. Heat for example, will always be directed away from the extremities to the core (abdomen,

chest, and brain area). Your hands and feet may get cold or freeze, but the body will send its last bit of heat to keep the core warm.

The body tends to keep toxins and salts in some type of storage solution instead of storing them as hard crystals or deposits. That is why if you have excess salt in your body, you may retain water. The body holds the water to keep the salt dissolved.

Your blood plasma is very similar in composition to sea water. Your blood needs to maintain a very precise specific gravity and pH. Simply put, the specific gravity is how heavy your blood is. Salt water weighs more than fresh water, it has a higher specific gravity. The saltier your body, the more water it needs to retain to keep the specific gravity where it should be. It has to grab water from all non-critical areas in the same manner the body grabs heat from non-critical areas. As you dump more salt into water, the greater its specific gravity (the heavier it becomes). The only way to bring the specific gravity down is to either get rid of some of the salt or add more water (dilute it). The only way to dilute the water is to get the water from somewhere. Guess where the water comes from. Either you drink more, or it pulls it from what is already there. When the body pulls it from itself, and remember, the human body is over 80 percent water, something has to dry out. The skin is the biggest organ and moist skin is not critical to life.

I use salt as an example, but the blood has many electrolytes, hormones and other chemicals in it. With our current environmental and dietary conditions, our blood has things in it that are just not meant to be there. So our body makes our skin drier so that our blood and other tissues can become wetter.

Second reason :

Toxins have a tendency to dry things out. When I fasted, the chemicals coming out through my breath were of a volatile nature. "Volatile" means they had a high vapor pressure or that they would evaporate rapidly. Rubbing alcohol is volatile. Drinking alcohol is volatile.

Drinking alcohol is used in many cosmetics when you want to get a fast drying effect. It is listed on the label as "SD" meaning specially denatured alcohol, the most common type being "SD40 alcohol." "Denaturing" means something has been added to the alcohol so that you cannot drink it. If you did, it would either make you very sick or kill you.

It has to be denatured or poisoned because there is no drinking alcohol tax paid on cosmetically used alcohol. You can drink alcohol until it destroys your liver, causes you to kill someone (60 percent of all homicides are committed under the influence of alcohol, not drugs), causes an auto accident, causes family violence (ask any battered woman if her husband was in**toxic**ated when he beat her, chances are it was alcohol), or causes a heart attack. But you cannot drink alcohol without paying the tax on it. For the love of money...

Alcohol evaporates quickly, making it ideal for cosmetics. Alcohol also carries fragrances well. When you splash on perfume or cologne, the alcohol evaporates quickly, and leaves the fragrance on your skin. Cosmetic alcohol is also much cheaper than pure oil based fragrances.

The major drawback with alcohol on the skin or hair is that alcohol dries them out. When alcohol goes on skin or hair, it dissolves whatever water or moisture it comes in contact with. When the alcohol evaporates, it takes the water with it, leaving the skin and hair drier.

I believe this phenomenon may be happening with a fast. As volatile chemical compounds are expelled from the body through the colon, urine, breath and skin, the compounds take water with them. I can't absolutely guarantee that this theory is correct, but I can guarantee that my skin did experience drying exactly as Mr. Gregory had predicted.

So what does that have to do with Jesus saying put some oil on your head? Remember I told you that I knew a lot about dry skin because of a product that I developed. I developed both a lotion and an oil that contain a total of 7 natural oils, and 14 natural herbal extracts.

I am not here to make a commercial for these products, but I do have a lot of confidence as well as many testimonials about them. The lotion is called MIRACLE LOTION® and the oil is called MIRACLE OIL®. Both suitable names from a preacher/chemist.

They are both available in many health food stores and beauty salons across the country. Many therapeutic massage therapists (not the massage parlor type) use MIRACLE OIL in their professional practice. MIRACLE LOTION was designed especially for dry skin of any type and particularly for those looking for a product that was as close to nature as possible and really worked.

In both products, only the best natural oils and herbs are used, so don't look for them in the 99¢ bin. As of this printing, Miracle Lotion® and Miracle Oil® sell for $9.00 per 8 oz. bottle.

Both products have a high natural oil content. A perfect blend of Olive Oil, Sweet Almond Oil, Canola Oil, Castor Oil, Safflower Oil, Sesame Seed Oil and Wheat Germ Oil are used.

The 14 herbs are Goldenseal, Comfrey, Cherry Bark, Chamomile, Hyssop, Sage, Sheep Sorrell, Henna, Black Walnut, Jaborandi, Wheat Germ, Alfalfa, Yarrow and Slippery Elm Bark.

I collaborated with an herbalist for the oil and herbal blend as well as the processing method because incorrect extraction or processing methods can kill the effectiveness of many natural ingredients. Improperly extracted herbs may be present in a product, but they are inactivated or "dead".

If your local health food store or beauty salon does not have MIRACLE OIL or MIRACLE LOTION, they can be ordered by calling 1-800-THE-WOMAN or online on the web at www.1800thewoman.com. **The Woman** stands for mother nature. The company accepts both Visa and MasterCard and the order lines are open 24 hours-a-day. Your health food store can order them for you to save you postage.

MIRACLE OIL and MIRACLE LOTION help minimize the drying of your skin during a fast. For a long fast, skin drying will probably happen both during and for a period of time after your fast.

Though Jesus meant the anointing of the head with oil for spiritual and ritual reasons, you do need to anoint your skin with oil or a very good lotion with a high oil content.

Many lotions have a high grease content. Products such as petrolatum and mineral oil are made from petroleum, the same source for gasoline and motor oil. They do not harm the body, and although many natural health experts speak against petroleum derived products, there is really nothing wrong with them. VASELINE® is pure petrolatum. Petrolatum and mineral oil are not as good for or absorbed as well by the skin as natural vegetable and plant oils. Petroleum oils are also much cheaper. That is why petroleum cosmetics are much cheaper to manufacture and sell. For a fast, I would use only the best and most natural ingredient products that I could find.

Also, MIRACLE OIL makes a super bath oil. Just a

tablespoon in your bath water will leave your skin feeling quite satiny. It also helps alleviate dry skin and the roughness that can occur during a fast.

That is one of the instructions for any fast that lasts five days or more. Keep your skin lubricated and moisturized with a GOOD product. There were several other instructions given in this verse in Matthew:

"But when you fast, put oil on your head and wash your face, so that it will not be obvious to men that you are fasting, but only to your Father, who is unseen; and your Father, who sees what is done in secret, will reward you."

The second instruction is perhaps the most important thing for you to do during your fast. If I had to list the things in order of importance, this would rank as #1.

Just as it is vitally important that you understand the FAST FLUSH and the M.E.S.S. toxins, it is equally important that you follow this instruction.

It cannot be overemphasized. It should **NEVER** be neglected. Dick Gregory told me that this was something that I should do daily. The books that I read all said that I should do this daily.

Do not laugh, frown, feel embarrassed or disgusted when I tell you what it is. At least listen as I explain why you MUST do this to get the maximum benefit from your fast. This is not something that most people will talk about.

I can understand that even if most ministers knew this, they would be reluctant to speak such words from the pulpit. I preached about it in a sermon one Sunday. The congregation laughed so hard until their sides hurt. It may sound funny, comedians often use this subject to make jokes about. No matter how it sounds, no matter how funny or disgusting, it's the truth and if you want your fast to give you the most benefit with the least amount of danger, you had better listen to this.

You can laugh until you cry. Laugh, but listen. Be disgusted, but obedient. Your life and health may depend on it.

Read about the most important thing you should do during your fast in the next chapter.

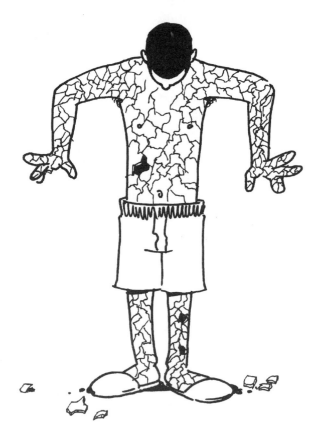

"Get yourself some oil because a long fast will cause your skin to dry out," said
Dick Gregory.

Chapter 11

WATER, WATER, WATER, EVERYWHERE

The first rule of fasting is simple. After you have properly gone through a good pre-fast regime you must put water, water, water everywhere.

Jesus said, *"wash your face, so that it will not be obvious to men that you are fasting,"*

The questions you might ask are, "What does washing your face have to do with men knowing that you are fasting?" "How are they going to know you are fasting just because you don't wash your face?" "Is my face going to get dirt on it from not eating?"

If it breaks out in a rash, washing will not remove the rash. If my face sinks in from loss of weight, washing will not restore that. From the surface, it appears that washing your face won't do anything to let people know that you are not fasting. All washing your face will do is give you a clean face.

What did Jesus mean by this? Many times when I am researching something in the Bible, I refer back to the Greek translation and the original Hebrew. If that does not explain it then I have to go back to the original language of Jesus, Aramaic.

The word "face" as used in the Bible is the Hebrew word "prosopon," defined as: the front (as being towards view), e.g., the countenance, aspect, appearance, surface; by implication— presence, person:(outward) appearance.

Interpretation from one language to another is always a little tricky. Idioms and slang terms may translate literally into something that was not meant at all.

For example, if a young person said, "that's a bad car you're driving" they actually mean that you are driving a good car, a nice looking car, an in-style car; a car that meets with their highest approval.

The literal translation of that, however, is that you are driving a "bad" or no good, raggedy, lemon of a car. The literal translation and the true meaning may be entirely different.

"Prosopon" may have meant face. It may have also meant the entire outside of the body. Again, the Greek definition of the word that "face" is also translated as the front (as being towards view), the countenance, aspect, appearance, surface; by implication- presence, person:--(outward) appearance.

Jesus could have very easily meant or said, "Wash your persona, your person, your outward appearance that men view."

If you walked among street-smart youth that regularly used vulgarity, and they felt that you needed a bath, they might use a vulgar statement such as, "you've got to go wash your a . ." or "your a . . is stinking".

They do not mean that your "a . ." or buttocks area is the only part that you need to wash. They mean you need to wash your whole body. The literal translation and what is often meant are two different things.

Jesus may have meant for them to wash their bodies, their whole person, so people would not know they were fasting. That makes sense. I am sure that even in the ancient days, they had M.E.S.S. toxins and the FAST FLUSH effect happened.

When they fasted, their bodies developed the same odors that ours do. It may have been even worse because they did not have hot daily showers, hot baths or deodorants as we do.

It became even more important for them to wash themselves if they were fasting and wanted to keep it secret. They would have to wash more than usual. They would have to wash their whole bodies. They would have to wash their mouths (or the face) because the M.E.S.S. would also be in the breath.

Fasting, unquestionably, causes a change in body odors. Sometimes the change is so drastic that even soap and hot water will not get rid of it and perfume or cologne will not cover it.

In the ancient days, people probably were not as toxic as we are today. They did not have the pesticides, the preservatives, the chemical additives, the hormones, the antibiotics, the drugs, and the pollution that surround us. Maybe plain soap and water would suffice for them.

This chapter is entitled, WATER, WATER, WATER EVERYWHERE. There are three types of water that are necessary during a fast. We have just talked about the first type, which utilizes cleansing water on the outside of the body. Believe it or not, this is the least important of the three. If you are alone, it becomes almost unimportant except that you have to be around yourself.

True to our nature in this narcissistic world, we would be more concerned about the water that washes the outside than any other. We often are not concerned how dirty our insides are, but we don't want others to see or smell a dirty outside.

Regardless of the smell or look, I recommend you keep your skin and mouth as clean as possible. The cleaner it is, the easier it is for the M.E.S.S. to come out. You can never go wrong by keeping something clean.

Washing our person during a fast has more meaning than just cleaning the outside.

The other two types of waters are the ones that are of vital importance. It is these that are the #1 thing that you must do during a fast. The rule is simple. . .

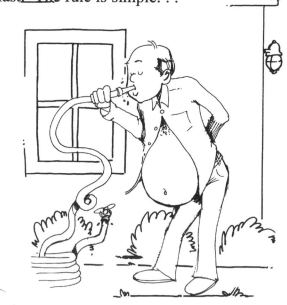

You MUST drink PLENTY of PURE WATER during your fast.
Water is essential to life. Water is essential to health. Clean water is essential to cleansing.

Chapter 12

You must put plenty of water in your body from both ends!

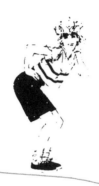

The top end:
You MUST drink PLENTY of PURE WATER during your fast. Water is essential to life. Water is essential to health. Clean water is essential to cleansing.

Remember this rule applies to anything in the world:

RULE:
IN ORDER TO MAKE SOMETHING CLEAN, YOU MUST ALSO MAKE SOMETHING DIRTY

Think of cleaning your house, clothes or car. You cannot clean any of them, without making something dirty. There is nothing dirty in the universe that you can clean without making something else dirtier.

Consider this:

◆ If you mop the floor, you make the mop and the mop water dirty.

◆ If you dust the furniture, you make the dust rag dirty.

◆ If you vacuum the carpet, you make the bag in the vacuum cleaner dirty.

◆ If you wash the dishes, you make the dishwater dirty.

◆ If you wash your car, you make rags and water dirty.

◆ If you take a bath, you leave a ring in the bath tub, while most of the dirt goes down the drain in dirty water headed on its way to make the sewer dirtier.

You cannot make something clean without making something else dirty. "What about if I sterilize it?" you ask. If you place something contaminated with germs on it under ultraviolet light or radiation, it will not make the light or the radiation dirty, that is true. But neither is anything being cleaned. Germs are being killed. The germs are still there, they are just DEAD. The law still applies. You can kill without being killed, but you cannot clean without something getting dirty.

Something
has to take away
and bear the dirt.

When you fast, that something that takes away and bears the dirt is WATER! You must pour plenty of water into your body from the top end. That means you must drink plenty of water.

You should drink 1/2 of your weight in water converted to ounces EVERY DAY whether you are fasting or not.

The original standard rule is that you should drink 8–8 oz. glasses of water every day. That rule is only a general average, but may not be correct for every person.

I will admit, if most people would drink 8 – 8 oz. glasses of water daily, it would be a vast improvement, but it may not be what they need for optimum health. I will explain why the 8 glass-a-day standard may not be right for you.

Science has long understood that medicines should be administered based on the condition and the SIZE of the person. The bigger a person (all other things being equal), the more medicine they need. Body weight makes a BIG difference in the effect of drugs, foods, alcohol and water.

If one person weighs 105 pounds and another weighs 285 pounds, common sense would tell you that they need different amounts of things (all other things being equal). I say "all other things being equal" because the small person could have a higher metabolism and actually burn up more food than the larger person, but this is usually more the exception than the rule.

Bigger people usually need more of anything material. They may be bigger for all the wrong reasons, but when it comes to water, bigger people need more water.

The 285 pound man or woman needs more water for their body to be at optimum health than the 105 pound person. This is just plain common sense. You do not need fancy studies to recognize this.

So the rule is not eight glasses of water a day. The rule is 1/2 your body weight converted in ounces per day. If you weigh 150 pounds, then you should drink 75 ounces of water a day. If you weigh 128 pounds, then you should drink 64 ounces of water daily, or 8 glasses. If you weigh 105 pounds, then you only need 53 ounces of water per day.

Body Weight in pounds divided by 2 equals

The amount of water you should drink daily in ounces

Your requirements may vary if you perform heavy exercises that cause water loss or if you live in extreme heat.

This is the rule for water intake when you are NOT fasting. Your intake of water should nearly DOUBLE when you fast.

Water does several things. First, it makes you feel full. Drinking water during a fast keeps the stomach full and reduces the feeling of hunger.

Second, it helps to flush the system of the M.E.S.S. toxins. Water is a good cleaner, and it is absolutely safe.

You must drink plenty of water during a fast.
This is the first half of the vital rule of fasting.

You should drink 75 to 100 percent of your body weight converted to ounces of water while you fast. If you weigh 200 pounds, then drink 150 to 200 ounces of water a day. That is a lot of water.

Do not take long automobile trips while your stomach is full of water. Do not get on small airplanes with no bathroom after you have just filled your stomach with water. Do not sit on a podium where you cannot leave several times if you have just filled your stomach with water.

When you drink that much water, you will probably need

um 20 glasses

to urinate quite often. That is one drawback to drinking your allotment of water. You have to use the rest room constantly. I get my allotment of water first thing in the morning. I drink a full 64 oz. of water. By 11 a.m., I have to use the rest room every 10 minutes. Either to urinate or to have a bowel movement.

You will be surprised what drinking your proper amount of water will do for constipation. Just try it for three days and see. I had a bathroom installed in my office. As I said, I value my health more than my car, and we have garages built for our cars don't we?

You might as well prepare for going to the bathroom a lot. You will also notice that the more water you drink, the less color and odor your urine will have.

Remember, as you fast, the FAST FLUSH process begins. Toxins flood into your bloodstream and tax all channels of elimination. Water poured into your system eases the burden on the other organs of elimination.

Imagine a very dirty car. It is caked with mud, dust and dirt. Now imagine that you are asked to clean it. You are given soap powder, a clean rag and tea cup of water. Tell me what is wrong with this picture.

That is the way your body is. Inside, it is caked with grime, buildup, M.E.S.S. and poison. The fast is the clean rag and the soap powder. It will scrub and lift the M.E.S.S. from your insides. It will cause the filth to be broken down and squeezed out of the tissues. The only problem is that you cannot clean a very dirty car with a small amount of water, no matter how many rags or how many boxes of soap powder you have.

YOU MUST HAVE AN ABUNDANCE OF WATER TO PROPERLY CLEAN THE VEHICLE!

The more water you drink, the faster and more thorough-ly the M.E.S.S. will be carried out of your body. The less water you drink, the more concentrated the loosened and squeezed out toxins will become.

THIS IS A PRIME AREA OF DANGER!
You MUST drink PLENTY of WATER!

Damage can result from the excess concentration of poi-sons. You must keep your body flowing with water. If it seems like I am overemphasizing this point–good. Water can make the difference between life or death, health or dis-ease, tragedy or triumph.

When you begin your fast, weigh yourself. You do not have to tell anyone your weight. If you weigh 250 pounds, that means you need to drink roughly one and a half to two gallons of water a day, (250 x 75% = 187 oz.; 250 x 100% = 250 oz). A gallon has 128 ounces, a quart has 32 ounces. Get two types of containers. The first type is a container large enough to hold your day's quota of water. The second type is a drinking container. If you need to drink one and a half to two gallons of water a day, first put your two gallons aside for that day.

You then need to schedule when and where you will drink your water. Get a LARGE glass or tumbler, say 32 oz. You then have to drink 6 to 8 - 32 oz. glasses to meet you allotment of water for the day. The bigger you are, the more water you can hold. The more water you drink, the greater the flushing effect.

Water cleans, water purifies, water restores, water soft-ens, water moisturizes and water deodorizes. You must get it in you for it to work.

182

12-16. 8oz glasses

The human body is 3/4 water, the same as the earth. You may spend an excessive amount of time running to the rest room, but you will restore and revitalize your body. Sometimes we just need a change of water.

That should be clear enough on that subject. If I have not said it loud enough I will repeat it again:

YOU MUST DRINK 75% TO 100% OF YOUR BODY WEIGHT IN OUNCES OF PURE WATER DURING YOUR FAST!!!

I just added one other thing. "PURE" water. During a fast you should not drink just ANY water, not even mineral water. There is only one type of water that you should drink during a fast.   RAIN WATER!

But what if you don't have any rain water?

Rain water goes by another name when it is man made. It is called "DISTILLED WATER". Distilled water is water that has been boiled and turned into steam. The steam is then cooled (technically called condensed) back into water. When water is turned into steam most of the impurities that are in the water are left behind as solids.

I said "most." There are still some organic compounds left that can still boil off. Therefore, distilled water is usually filtered to remove any last traces of impurities.

You can buy distilled water at most grocery stores. It is better to buy it in glass bottles, but glass has become almost impossible to find. Storing water in plastic, especially the thinner cheap plastic has a tendency to flavor the water.

Sears sells an excellent water distiller for home use. It is not cheap, but it is excellent. It makes a gallon of freshly distilled water in 6 to 8 hours, and it has a charcoal filter. This may be an expensive alternative since a gallon of distilled water in the grocery store is under $2. Again we have to ask ourselves, would I spend that much to fix up my car?

There is a reason for using distilled water. Spring water or mineral water may not have the harmful impurities that tap water has, however, they are not preferred for a fast. Distilled water has absolutely nothing in it. It is as pure as you can get for water.

Mineral water may contain sodium, which more than likely your body has an excess of. It probably needs to get rid of some. Mineral water may contain many other minerals that will act as food for a fasting body. It may slow the fasting process if you are on a pure water fast.

The only thing the experts allow in the water is the juice of a freshly squeezed lemon. You take one gallon of distilled water and add the juice of one lemon. Add NO SWEETEN-ER, just the juice of one lemon. No sugar, no honey, no Nutrasweet®, just the juice of one lemon per gallon of distilled water. Do not use store bought lemon juice. Use the juice of a freshly squeezed lemon.

Why lemon juice?

This gets a little complicated. It has to do with the pH of the M.E.S.S. toxins, the proper pH of the bloodstream, the metabolizing of the lemon and its neutralizing qualities. I am tempted to skip explaining this, but I won't. I want you to completely understand what you are doing. I do not want to just tell you to do something without explaining why. You have a right to know, and I have a responsibility to tell you.

Your blood plasma is virtually identical to sea water. The plasma is what is left without the cells. It is a clear or yellowish fluid. When hemoglobin-rich red blood cells are added to blood plasma, then you have red blood.

The pH of the blood in its correct state is slightly alkaline, just like sea water. It has a pH in the average person of 7.35 to 7.45. The pH scale is a logarithmic scale, just like the Richter scale for earthquakes. A logarithmic scale means that each number unit difference represents a factor of 10, not 1.

For example, an earthquake that measures 6 on the Richter scale is 10 times stronger than one that measures 5, and 100 times stronger than one that measures 4. Each unit represents 10 times the difference either up or down from the next unit.

pH (which technically means the inverse logarithm of the hydronium ion concentration) is simply a measure of how acid or alkaline something is. Pure distilled water has a pH of 7.0. Anything below 7 is considered an acid, anything above 7 is considered an alkali or a base.

Blood is an alkali because it has a pH above 7 (7.35 to 7.45). For good health, blood must be kept at the proper pH. If you have ever owned a marine aquarium (yes, I have one), you know the importance of keeping the pH at the proper level. Salt water fish are extremely sensitive to changes in pH. To the fish, the water is their blood. It performs virtually the same functions as the blood in our bodies. If the aquarium pH drifts tremendously, the fish get sick and die. If our blood pH drifts tremendously, we get sick and die.

Things that we take into our bodies are metabolized and waste products are produced. Drugs (most illegal, and many legal drugs) are in a class called alkaloids. They are alkali in nature, but when they are metabolized in the body they turn into an acid waste product.

Many foods turn into acid waste products. Acid waste products reduce the pH of the blood and make it more acidic.

The more acidic it gets, the more unhealthy we become, and the more that happens, the closer we get to death.

Lemons are acid fruits, but when metabolized in the body, they turn into an alkali. They increase the pH of the blood. The M.E.S.S. toxins are acids in the body and the bloodstream. The alkali metabolite of the lemon juice helps to neutralize the acid of the M.E.S.S. and helps in the elimination and cleansing process.

Do not ask me about oranges, grapefruits or tangerines. Use just one lemon per gallon of distilled water. One fresh lemon that is fresh squeezed.

We have covered the water of the external washing. We have covered the water of the internal washing from the top end. Remember, I said from both ends. I hear you screaming, "But there is only one other end!" Guess what, "You've got to wash out your. . ."

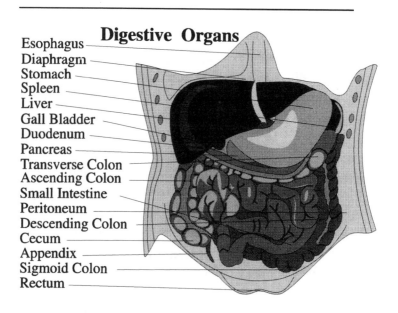

Digestive Organs

Esophagus
Diaphragm
Stomach
Spleen
Liver
Gall Bladder
Duodenum
Pancreas
Transverse Colon
Ascending Colon
Small Intestine
Peritoneum
Descending Colon
Cecum
Appendix
Sigmoid Colon
Rectum

Chapter 13

STUCK UP
AND
BLOWN AWAY

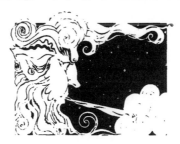

This is the second part of the most vital thing you MUST do during a fast. You must take an enema every day. DON'T LAUGH and don't stop reading. **THIS IS IMPORTANT!**

We do not like to talk about going to the bathroom to defecate. Only comedians of the grossest type use bathroom humor. We are embarrassed about it. A husband and wife can be married for 50 years and experienced many intimate situations together.

They can share sexual secrets and fantasies that would shock their children. They may have very few secrets, but there is one area where they are alone and do not share.

Whenever they have to do a #2, defecate, boo boo, BM, or a host of other names, it becomes a completely private matter. In men's rooms, urinals are usually out in the open. A man will stand hip to hip with another man and urinate.

Yet the stalls where #2 takes place are not only closed in, but they have locks on the doors. Why do we need locks on the door?

When we are sitting on the commode, we feel embarrassed and powerless. We want no other human being to be in our "boo boo" space. How often and when we boo boo is a closely guarded secret. It is taboo.

The technical name for it is "Bowel Movement." Most of us have called it BM from the time we were children. So, that's what I will use, "BM."

Let's become mature, unlock the door and talk about BMing. There is nothing to be ashamed of. If you are sitting somewhere in public reading this book, look over at the person nearest you. No matter how rich they are, no matter how well dressed or how well educated or sophisticated, that rich, sophisticated person BM's just like you do.

If they do not BM, you will not see them around for very long.

The colon is an organ of elimination. Our entire digestive system is essentially one long tube. Your mouth is on one end of the tube and your anus is on the other end (the anus is the hole that your BM comes out of). At least you cannot say that I did not thoroughly explain things to you. BM, (the solid stuff), is called "feces." The "bowel movement" refers to the act of defecating, not the "solid stuff," but I think it is clear what we are talking about. There is no need for overly technical terms, "BM" will suffice for describing the act and the solid stuff.

The tube with your mouth on one end and your anus on the other (technically called the alimentary canal), is more than 20 feet long. Some people have a greater distance between their mouth and their anus than others. That's both a physical and a philosophical statement.

The tube or alimentary canal consists of four basic parts:

1. **The Pharynx** - The section of the alimentary canal that extends from the mouth and nasal cavities to the larynx, where it becomes continuous with the esophagus.
2. **The Esophagus** - The muscular, membranous tube for the passage of food from the pharynx to the stomach.
3. **The Stomach** - a saclike principal organ of digestion.
4. **The Intestines** -The portion of the Alimentary Canal from the stomach to the anus, consisting of the small and large intestine.

We often take our digestive system for granted. Again, go to the drug or grocery store and look at the shelves. Look at the laxatives and at digestion aids. Notice how filled the shelves are with antacids, the pink stuff, stuff for coating stomachs, stuff for diarrhea and stuff for gas.

Our digestive system is serious business. Heart disease is the No. 1 killer in this country. The bypass operation is the leading operation. You get your heart bypassed because the vessels are clogged up with M.E.S.S. Call it cholesterol or plaque or whatever name you choose. It is still M.E.S.S.

Heart disease is No. 1 and cancer is No. 2. The National Center for Health Statistics cites the leading form of cancer is CANCER OF THE DIGESTIVE SYSTEM. Respiratory (lung) cancer ranks behind digestive system cancer. Guess where the most digestive system cancer occurs. It's in the colon. There is death in the colon of most Americans. For women, colon cancer is the second leading cause of cancer deaths, right behind breast cancer.

Television ads show women how to examine breasts for breast cancer. Yet, for women, colon cancer is immediately behind breast cancer. Shouldn't we examine our colons?

Digestion of food begins in the mouth, the beginning end of the alimentary canal or digestive tract. Food is chewed and mixed with saliva which contains the enzyme ptyalin (amylase) which breaks down starch. Food leaves the mouth, travels through the esophagus to the stomach. Once in the stomach, the stomach lining secretes gastric juice that contains hydrochloric acid and various enzymes. The enzyme pepsin begins protein digestion, lipase speeds the hydrolysis of certain fats, rennin (in infants) curdles milk.

The stomach has a churning motion that breaks food into tiny particles while mixing the food with gastric juice. The liquid food called chyme then enters the duodenum (the beginning portion of the small intestine). Solid food remains in the stomach until it liquifies (usually 1 to 6 hours).

Some absorption of water, alcohol and drugs occurs in the stomach, but chyme passes mostly unabsorbed into the duodenum. Most digestion and absorption occur in the small intestine.

The surface of the small intestine is covered by a mucous membrane that contains millions of villi. Villi are small hair like projections that wave like wheat in the wind. For digestion, numerous enzymes enter the small intestines produced by the intestinal lining and the pancreas.

Pancreatic enzymes include trypsin, which breaks down protein into its individual amino acids; lipase, which breaks down fats to fatty acids and glycerol; and amylase, which breaks down starches to sugars.

Intestinal enzymes include erepsin, which also breaks down proteins to amino acids; lactase, maltase and sucrase, which breaks down complex sugars. A deficiency in lactase results in the inability to properly break down lactose (milk sugar) and gives people gas and other difficulty when they drink milk or eat some milk products. Finally, enterkinase is secreted, which activates trypsin.

Bile is secreted by the liver which helps neutralize stomach acid and aids the small intestine to emulsify and absorb fats and fat soluble vitamins. Emulsify means to dissolve fatty stuff (fats and oils) into water based solutions.

When the food reaches the point where the small intestine joins the large intestine, virtually all the nutritional value has been absorbed.

The large intestine is called large intestine because it is actually much larger in diameter than the small intestine. The large intestine primarily absorbs water from the remaining material and stores the residual stuff before passing it out during a BM.

This was a brief summary of what happens to your food once you put it in your mouth. At least this was what is SUPPOSED to happen once you put the food in your mouth. Unfortunately, it does not usually work out that way.

First, we often fail to thoroughly chew our food. Many foods will not properly digest if not thoroughly chewed. If the initial enzyme, Ptyalin, is not allowed to begin the digestive process, the food will not be properly digested.

We are often in a hurry. We not only order fast food but we eat it fast. Food should be chewed until it is virtually a liquid before you swallow it. The professional advice is this, "You should drink your food and chew your liquid."

You should chew your food so thoroughly that you practically drink it. This helps to ensure, even with "bad foods" that the digestion process will continue. This does not mean that you drink along with your food. Health experts all say that you should not drink ANYTHING, not even water, with your food. When you drink while eating, you dilute the digestive juices and reduce the efficiency and completeness of your digestion.

You should chew your liquids. Chewing your liquids refers to swishing the liquid in your mouth to thoroughly mix the liquids with saliva before drinking it. Just as solid foods require digestion, so do liquids (other than water). Liquids are foods too, and they have to be broken down, digested and absorbed. When you chew your liquids, you allow the digestion to begin in the mouth.

Second, we hinder digestion when we eat the wrong combination of foods. We generally think nothing of eating six to 10 foods at a meal. We never stop to think if all of these foods are going to digest well together. There is a good probability that they do not.

In the brief lesson above, you learned the stomach secretes an acid. An acid is what is needed to digest a protein. But an acid is not what is needed to digest a starch. An alkali, which is the OPPOSITE of an acid, is what is needed to digest a starch.

So what happens when you eat a protein and a starch together? It sits in your stomach for hours on end trying to get digested. Proteins and starches just do not digest well together. It's a great deal for the drug companies. They get to sell you millions of dollars of antacids as you try to recover from dumping all of that acid in your stomach. You are trying to digest starch when the starch is hollering for an alkaline solution.

What are proteins and starches? Meat and potatoes, bread and meat, spaghetti and meatballs and even fish and chips. But these are American standards! I know they are. But the American gut is in a mess. Or shall I say shall the American gut is filled with M.E.S.S.

Isn't a potato a vegetable? Yes, if you eat it raw or steamed. When you bake it or fry it, it becomes a pasty starch.

The principles of proper food combining will do wonders for your digestion, energy and weight. It is not complicated or hard to do. Again, I suggest that you get the book, FIT FOR LIFE. It will thoroughly explain and tell you all you need to know about how to eat to prevent colon cancer and an upset stomach. You only need to read Part 1, which is only 137 pages, to learn all that you need to know.

This may sound like another commercial like MIRACLE OIL ® and MIRACLE LOTION ®, but these are products that will make a change in your life.

Get the book FIT FOR LIFE!

When we eat fast, eat the wrong combination, eat the wrong foods, our food does not get properly digested. What happens when it is not properly digested?

There are ONLY TWO THINGS THAT CAN HAPPEN. The undigested food is either eliminated, or it stays in us. Some of both happens depending upon whose system it is. Some comes out, and some stays in. When it stays in, it cakes up in the digestive tract. Often, it stays caked up until the person dies, festering and decaying in 100 degree, moist heat.

Estimates by fasting experts suggest that the average person has between 5 to 35 pounds of caked up, blackened, hardened, rotting, undigested food in their colon and digestive tract.

I heard this over and over as I read about it in books on fasting. I heard about it as I attended The Natural Hygiene Seminars, but I did not believe that it was true about me.

I did not believe it for several reasons.

I eat correctly. By correctly, I mean that I eat very healthy. Since I was 17, and attended the first Natural Hygiene Convention, my diet has been fairly pure. I ate very little meat and dairy products. I ate an abundance of fresh fruits and steamed vegetables. My body was slim, I had no potbelly, my stomach was like the proverbial washboard. I exercised regularly. I never used drugs (legal or illegal), smoked cigarettes or consumed alcohol.

I did not have any of the classic signs that would indicate any caked up M.E.S.S. in my digestive tract. When I decided to go on a fast, Dick Gregory gave me another bit of advice, he said, "make sure that you take an enema **EVERY DAY**."

He explained that the poisons that would come out of my system must be flushed out or they could poison my system. I did not believe him. I had fasted many times before and had never taken an enema, and I did not have any problems, why did I need one now? I believed that it was true that "other folk" were caked up, but not me because I was clean.

After I had been on my fast for three days, I decided that I would try an enema. I had never taken an enema before. I did not think it was necessary for me because I had been on The Eden Diet for nine days before I started my fast.

I was in Hollywood, Florida. I had gone to the ocean for my fast. I had started fasting in the winter, so it was a good idea to be in warm weather during the fast.

I had to first find the enema equipment. Most drug stores only had the little 8 oz. plastic squeeze jar with the nozzle on it. It came with a pre-filled solution in the jar. That will not work!

For an enema on a fast, you need a real enema, not the little squeeze jar. You need a MINIMUM of a 1500 ml enema bag. Enema bags generally come in two sizes, a 1500 ml or a two quart bag. Either will do, but the two quart bag is better.

I found two types of nozzles. They both look very similar but with one major difference. One type of nozzle has a hole only at the tip, the other type has a hole at the tip and one on the side about a half an inch behind the tip.

If you can find it, get the type with the two hole nozzle, it works MUCH better than the one hole type.

Also, a transparent bag is better. A see-through bag does not work any different, but you can visually see when the water is out of the bag. Taking an enema is simple once you are used to it.

When I took my first enema I was shocked. I thought that my colon was clean, especially since I had been on The Eden Diet for nine days, and I had a BM for every meal that I ate. This description may get a little gross, but a BM is not known for its fragrant appeal.

After the first enema I looked into the commode. It was a full bowel movement. The commode was full of feces. The feces was normal. "Boy," I thought, "I had a full BM still in me, well at least that's all out now."

I reasoned that I still had a full colon since there was no new food to push the last food out. There is one thing that happened after the first enema and continued to happen after each enema. You feel great after an enema.

The next day I decided to take another enema, "just to see" if anything else was left. Was I surprised! Not only was there plenty left, but it was not normal feces. It was horrible, and there was plenty of it!

It was black and very smelly. My feces (BM) normally does not have much odor. This stuff was foul! I took an enema that morning and another that night. Both times, stuff poured out. It was stringy, like bits of seaweed, only it was jet black and it stank to high heaven.

I became an instant believer in the necessity of daily enemas. During that entire fast, I took an enema in the morning, and an enema before I went to sleep. Each time the horrible stuff poured out. "When is this stuff going to stop coming out?" I wondered.

Although it was very gross, the scientist in me was amazed. How could this much stuff possibly be in me? I was so-called "clean." Day after day, enema after enema, it poured out. I estimate that at least one to two pounds of M.E.S.S. came out of me each day.

Because I had studied much about fasting, I knew what was happening, I just could not believe it was happening to me. Trust me on this. You will see it for yourself when you PROPERLY go on your fast.

YOU HAVE AT LEAST 5 TO 35 POUNDS OF JUNK CAKED UP INSIDE OF YOU AND IT IS ROTTING MORE AND MORE EACH DAY

This is not being boastful, just honest. If I had that much in me, and I eat virtually none of the things that clog you up, imagine what the average American has.

While on the fast I went out to the beach. People were strolling constantly along the boardwalk. Seventy five percent of the men over 35 had one thing in common. They had potbellies. Most had rather significant potbellies, beer guts or whatever you want to call them. A significant majority had major potbellies.

As I took my enemas, I could not help wondering. If my stomach is flat as a board and this much is coming out of me, **what is in those big potbellies?** The thought of that made me shiver.

We are a nation that is rapidly becoming poisoned from the inside. Bloated bellies are a sign of either starvation, malnutrition or clogged undigested food malnutrition.

No wonder colon cancer is the second leading cancer and will probably get much worse. If you saw what came out of me, and imagined that still inside you, you would make an immediate effort to get it out of you.

I could easily see how such an internal cesspool could cause cancer. That kind of M.E.S.S. sitting for years on end in your gut has to cause some problems. I just could not get over what came out of me, but I was glad that it did.

Each time I saw the commode blackened and stinking, I knew that something was being made clean and something was being made dirty. The sewer system was being made dirtier, but my system was being made cleaner.

On the seventh day of the fast, I went to Hallendale Florida to get a colonic. I had to call around to find a colonic clinic nearby, and I found one. There was so much stuff still coming out that I needed to get something to get that M.E.S.S. out of me even faster.

A colonic or colonic irrigation is really a high powered enema. A technician lays you on a table and inserts the tube into your anus. Water is then pumped into you just like the enema. The technician does this over and over, sometimes for over an hour until they think the colon is clean.

The technician ran water in and out of me for 30 to 40 minutes until the water ran almost clear. The water at the end had a slight yellowish cast to it. "That's bile from your liver detoxifying," the technician said. I had informed them that I was fasting and that was why I wanted a colonic.

"Is this everything in me?" I asked. "That was it," the technician said. "Everything should be out of you now, you will not need to take any more enemas," the technician responded.

During the 25 to 30 times the technician ran water in and out of me, I could see the M.E.S.S. coming out through the clear tube. The tech said it was mucus and feces coming out. The technician would massage my stomach to manipulate the colon and physically break up M.E.S.S. that was there. I also did this during my enemas.

A colonic costs anywhere from $50 to $75. Most cities have several colonic clinics. The quality of the technicians will vary as with anything else. How long it will take when you get a colonic will depend upon how clogged you are.

When I arrived back at my motel room, I was relieved that I had all the M.E.S.S. removed from my system.

The next evening, I decided to take one more enema just to make sure everything was out. Guess what? Stuff still poured out. Awful, ugly, stinking stuff and piles of it, poured out.

I then realized why fasting and enemas were so necessary. The M.E.S.S. inside you is caked up. It is hardened like baked on mud. When you fast, your body devotes its energy to breaking down and removing the junk. It did not get in there in a few days, it took decades. It will not come out in a few days.

The colonic did not get all the M.E.S.S. out because the colonic could only remove the loose M.E.S.S. Much of the M.E.S.S. was still in the hardened form and was slowly being broken loose layer by layer. A colonic is good, but it will in no way replace the daily enema or enemas.

I took two enemas a day, approximately 12 hours apart. I took an enema at 9 or 10 in the morning and one at 9 or 10 at night. Each time, a load of M.E.S.S. came out. You may not believe that there is that much in you. I know I did not. But believe me, it is there, and it needs to come out.

All the M.E.S.S. is not in the colon. When you fast, the body cleans itself out. M.E.S.S. from every organ, from stored toxic fat deposits, M.E.S.S. from all parts of the body is flushed out and into the colon. Fasting is the only way to get it out. And you must take enemas.

During my first 7-day fast, I did not take an enema and I had no BM's after the first day. Many people do experience a BM every day while fasting, but that is probably because they were highly constipated in the first place.

I think back on how much M.E.S.S. was left in my system because I failed to take the daily enemas. You may have your doubts about what I am telling you. I will tell you two words in answer to your skepticism. TRY IT! Try it and see.

It will not cost you a thing. It will actually save you money on food. For seven days try this simple plan.

For the first three days, go on The Eden Diet. For the last four days go on a full water fast. Take an enema daily during the full fast and see what happens. You may be even more surprised than I was.

A note of caution: Enemas can be too depleting and strenuous for some elderly fasters although many elderly use enemas regularly as a laxative. Once you have removed the caked up M.E.S.S. from your system, enemas will be less beneficial and **usually unnecessary** for a fairly clean system on subsequent fasts.

Enemas have their greatest benefit for the initial removal of the years of caked up, hardened, and blackened deposits that exist in the vast majority of adult westerners.

Now that you know that you must take an enema until you clean out the hardened M.E.S.S. while you fast, you must also know how to properly take an enema. The instructions follow in the next chapter.

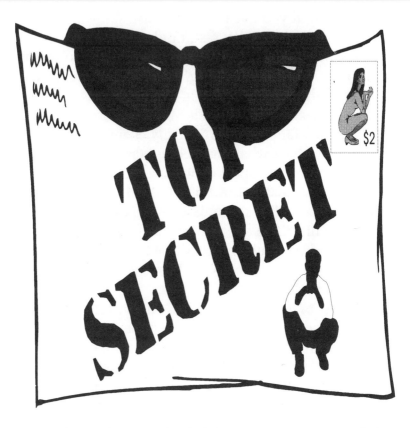

Whenever they have to do a #2, defecate, boo boo, BM, or a host of other names, it becomes a completely private matter. In men's rooms, the urinals are usually out in the open. A man will stand hip to hip with another man and urinate. Yet the stalls where #2 takes place are not only closed in, but they have locks on the doors. Why do we need a lock on the door?

Chapter 14

HOW TO
PROPERLY
TAKE AN ENEMA

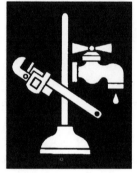

First you need the proper equipment. You need at least a 1500 ml (about 1 1/2 quarts) preferably a two quart enema bag. Enema bags are usually sold as a combination enema/douche kit. The bag is the same, the only difference is the nozzle. One type is used for douching the vagina and another type is used for an enema.

If you can find it, get the type of enema nozzle that has two holes in it, one at the tip and one on the side behind the tip. I bought this type from the colonic irrigation clinic. Surprisingly, it was a better unit and it was less than half of the cost of the unit from the drug store.

You will need some fresh lemons or brown vinegar, a piece of thin cloth for straining the lemon juice, a plastic gallon jug, and some lubricant for placing the nozzle in your anus. Do not use petroleum-based products. You may use either natural oil-based products, (MIRACLE OIL works great for this), pure Olive Oil, or a water soluble lubricant.

You must first prepare the water solution. Fill the plastic jug with lukewarm water. The water should be around body temperature (95º to 100ºF). Do not have the water too hot. You cannot hold the water in you very long when it is too hot.

Cut the lemon in half, place the cloth over one half and squeeze the juice into the jug. Repeat for the other half. You may use either lemon juice (best) or brown vinegar (second best) but you do not need both. If you use vinegar, add 2-4 tablespoons of vinegar. Mix the lemon juice or the vinegar in the jug.

Place the enema bag about two to three feet above the floor in your bathroom. Hooking the enema bag on the doorknob is usually about the right height. The higher the bag is above you, the stronger the flow of water. You do not want the flow too strong. Often the discomfort of an enema comes from two areas. The water is either too hot or cold, or the bag is too high and the water flows too hard.

The bag must be placed at a point where the tube can easily reach your anus when you are laying flat on the floor. You can set up your bag on the bathroom floor, in the shower or in the bathtub. You may use STRONG clothes hangers to lower the enema bag from the curtain rod to a point 2-3 feet above you.

Enema bags come with a clamp that fits over the tube near the nozzle end. Clamp the tube shut. Fill the bag with your warm water solution to the fill line on the bag. You will still have half of the solution left. I recommend that you repeat each enema twice at each session.

Place the jug on the floor and place the nozzle in the jug.

Open the clamp and let about one half cup of the water flow into the jug from the bag. This removes all the air from the line. You only want water going in you. You do not need air in there. There is probably enough gas there already.

Place some lubricant on the nozzle. Use your finger to place some lubricant around your anus. You do not need much, just enough to make it slippery.

Place a towel over the spot where you will lie flat.

You are now ready to begin:

Lie on your LEFT SIDE, not your right, always start an enema on your LEFT SIDE. There is a good reason for this. I had to look at an anatomical diagram of the intestines to understand why you need to start an enema on your left side.

The colo-rectal tube does not go straight up from your anus. It makes a 90° turn to the left and then goes up the left side of the body, then it crosses over and goes down the right side of the body *(see page 136)*. If you started an enema on your right side, the water could not go beyond the first few inches. Imagine placing a horseshoe against your stomach with the open end facing down. Now imagine a tube running from your anus to the LEFT end of the horseshoe. That's about how your colo-rectal tube is made. That is why you MUST start an enema on your left side.

ALWAYS START AN ENEMA
LAYING ON YOUR *LEFT* SIDE

While laying on your left side, gently insert the nozzle from the enema bag into your anus. The instructions with the bag will indicate how far to place the nozzle in your anus. Usually two to three inches is as far as it needs to go.

Open the clamp on the nozzle and let the water flow. The first time you take an enema, the water flowing is a rather odd experience. You become used to it after a few times.

As the water flows in, gently BUT FIRMLY, massage your abdomen where the colon is. This does two things. It helps to break up and release the M.E.S.S. as the water flows in. It also releases trapped air as the water flows in. As the water flows in, air is displaced.

Constantly massage your abdomen. If you have a transparent bag, turn on your back after 1/3 of the water has gone in. If you do not have a see-through bag you have to estimate when 1/3 of the water has gone in.

Continue to massage your abdomen while on your back. After another 1/3 of the water has gone in, turn on your right side.

Continue to massage your abdomen while on your right side. After all of the water has gone in, massage your abdomen while turning from your right side, to your back, to your left side.

Remember, the water is washing the inside of a dirty tube. You should try to let the water stay in you for 10 to 15 minutes. You may not be able to hold the water in that long. Often the urge to BM becomes urgent after the water has gone in.

When you stand up to BM, shake your stomach from side to side, back and forth, and round and round. You will hear the water sloshing inside you. Imagine a washing machine because that is what is happening inside. The more you can shake and slosh the water, the more cleaning you get, and the more M.E.S.S. you will break loose. Do not get too vigorous with the shaking if you are not in shape for it. I would not want you to throw your back out of kilter.

Some suggest that you should just lie there while the water is in you and move from the left side to your back, then to the right side. I don't think so. If you are trying to remove

M.E.S.S., you need several things to speed it up.

You need a cleaning agent, (water and the lemon juice) and you need contact time. The longer the water is in contact with the M.E.S.S., the softer and easier to remove it gets.

You need mechanical action. Mechanical action is simply scrubbing. When you move and slosh the water, it scrubs. It is the same as a washing machine agitator. When you wash clothes you have a pre-soak cycle, but the sloshing is where the cleaning takes place. Lie there and pre-soak, but slosh to get the M.E.S.S. out.

You also need to slosh while lying down. Remember the colon is shaped like a horseshoe and you must make sure the water gets to the right side, not just the left side. While lying on your back, raise your hips and slosh. That will help the water get evenly distributed throughout the colon.

Hold the water for 10 to 15 minutes or for as long as you can if you can't hold it 10 to 15 minutes. After the time is up or either you can't hold the water any longer, you are ready to BM.

Now I am going to tell you how to properly BM.

I can hear you saying, "I may not know a lot about fasting, but I know how to BM. I have been BMing all of my life." I know you have been BMing all of your life, but you probably have not been BMing properly.

Again, look at your pets. When they have a BM, what do they do? Do they sit on a toilet? No. They do not have a toilet. Even if you provided a kitty or doggie toilet, they would not use it. Why? **Because they are not supposed to sit while they BM and neither are you!**

Look at the diagram of the colon. The colon is a tube. When you sit, the tube is chinked. You know what happens when you put a kink in a water hose. The water stops flowing or at least it slows down a lot. Eighty percent of all colon cancers occur in the spots where the kinks are.

Most people in primitive countries do not have toilets, but they BM properly because they squat. Squatting straightens out the tube and allows proper contraction of the muscles that assists in BMing. That is how your cat or dog defecates. They squat. So should you.

Not only will it reduce your chances of colon cancer, but you will eliminate much more without the kinks in the tube. Don't take my word for it. **TRY IT!**

How can you squat on a commode? You can't practically, but you can imitate the same relative positioning and muscle tension as squatting. I own a device that helps you. It is really nothing but a raised step that you place your feet on while sitting on the commode (called the Welles Step). It works great and The Welles Step is very simple to use.

You can duplicate it very easily. If you have phone books, you can use those. You will need two sets of phone books that are eight to ten inches high. Any type of books will work. Two small boxes will work or anything where you can SECURELY place both feet while sitting on the toilet that is eight to 10 inches high.

Place the phone books (or whatever) on the floor where you normally place your feet while sitting on the toilet. Sit on the toilet. Place your feet on the phone books. Make sure the books are steady. I don't want you falling off the toilet. Bend your head forward to where your head is over your knees and place about 1/3 of your weight on your feet.

This sounds complicated, but it is quite comfortable. Now go on and BM.

If you do not have any phone books available or if you have to BM in someone else's rest room, there is again a simple but effective way to imitate the correct squatting position. This is my own invention, but it really works. It is quick and easy and requires no devices, books or boxes. Don't associate this with the name "Bronner." I don't want this to be called "The Bronner Maneuver." Although if people employed this technique it would save lives and reduce illnesses, I still would rather my name not be attached to it. I can imagine a large sporting event, a man gets up, his friends ask him "Where is he going?" "I am going to do a Bronner Maneuver," he replies. I would rather be famous for something else.

When sitting on the toilet, do two things: *(see pic. pg. 138)*
1. Bend your head forward and down to the position where your head is between your knees. Your back should be as close to parallel to the floor as possible. Your shoulders should touch your knees. Grab your legs between your ankle and knee. Grab your left leg with your left hand and your right leg with your right hand.

2. Pull your shoulders down against your knees and BM.

That's it. By bending forward and placing your head between your knees you effectively straighten the tube out. By pulling your shoulders down you cause muscles to contract that aid in elimination.

You will feel the difference this position makes. You may notice that up to **TWICE AS MUCH** BM comes out this way. Not only does more come out, it comes out faster and easier. You should ALWAYS BM like this. **NEVER BM sitting straight up on a toilet.**

You eliminate faster, with less strain, and you eliminate more in this correct position. This is the next best thing to squatting. Now you know **HOW** to BM properly.

This information alone will be worth hundreds, thousands or tens of thousands of times the price that you paid for this book. When your colon is clean, you feel better and have less chance of all diseases. This maneuver, helps to keep your colon clean.

After you have taken the first enema, and had a BM, repeat the exact same procedure with the remainder of the water in the jug. You will usually find that you cannot hold as much water the second time as the first. You may need to go through the procedure several times to get the entire gallon of water in and out of you.

You feel different after a good enema. Your body knows that it has just eliminated a pile of toxic waste, and you will feel the difference.

Make sure that you keep the nozzle well lubricated with a good lubricant. The enemas are not harmful but your anus could become irritated if proper lubrication is not used for the nozzle.

To sum up WATER, WATER, WATER, EVERYWHERE.

The first water is the washing of the external body. It is the least important but good for personal hygiene and to allow the skin to rid the body of many poisons.

The second water is to drink 75 to 100 percent of your body weight in pounds converted to ounces of distilled water each day. You may add the freshly squeezed juice of one lemon per gallon of water.

The third water is to take at least one enema per day, with a minimum of a 1500 ml enema bag. Use lemon juice or brown vinegar in the enema water. Slosh the water well when it is in you. Always use the **proper** squatting position when you BM.

ADDITIONAL QUESTIONS AND ANSWERS

Q: ***What about exercising while I Fast?***

A: **All things in moderation.** I exercise EVERY day when I fast. Believe it or not, exercising gives me energy. The major complaint during fasting is often lack of energy. Exercising stimulates my system, and I usually feel better after exercising.

There are numerous reports of fasters walking or running great distances while on a long fast. Usually, the energy increases after the second week of fasting, after the bulk of the toxins has been eliminated. The fasters that perform those feats are not the average fasters. They usually have fasted many times before, and their bodies are somewhat used to it. They also are usually in very good shape when they start their fast.

There is, however, an opposite school of thought. Many fasting clinics will not even allow patients to get out of bed during a long fast. They believe the patient should allow ALL of their energy to be focused on the cleansing and healing process. Experts opinions vary on this question, but my personal experience is that exercising during a fast is beneficial.

The answer to this question also depends upon the type of

exercise you have in mind and what physical condition you were in before you started fasting.

If you jogged 10 miles per week before you began your fast, you could easily briskly walk five miles per week during your fast. If two flights of steps tired you out before your fast, and you were not in the habit of exercising, five miles of brisk walking would be a very bad idea for you.

Exercise is individual. Under no circumstances should you do more during a fast than you regularly did before your fast. Getting in shape comes in stages.

If you are completely out of shape and suddenly begin to exercise, it tears your body down. You may get aches and pains, become sore and get tremendously out of breath. But then the body will begin to rebuild.

I occasionally lift weights. If I have not lifted for a very long time and I suddenly start to lift weights again, I will lose weight during the first week of my workout. After the first week, I continually gain weight and put on muscle. That first week tears down the body before the rebuilding starts.

If you are completely out of shape, a fast is no time to try to build something (like muscle). If you are in great shape, a reduced program from your current exercise program will be fine. Exercise depends upon the individual, and the physical condition that they are in.

I would recommend that everyone on a fast also exercise. The only differences are the types and degrees of exercising. If you are not in very good shape, then walking or stretching are the only types of exercises you should do on a fast.

Exercising also speeds up the detoxifying process because movement squeezes toxins out and increases circulation. Circulation is what carries the toxins out of and away from the tissues. Many rashes and bumps can appear during exercising on a fast because the activity causes the toxins to be released at an accelerated rate.

I always exercise on a fast, but I exercise even when I am not fasting. I use a reduced exercise program, nothing muscle building, only walking, light jogging and stretching.

This answer also depends upon how long you are fasting. The longer the fast, generally, the less strenuous the exercise. Also it depends upon how much fat you have. The fatter you are, the more fuel and toxins your body will have to burn during the fast.

Generally you should follow these guidelines:

◆ You should exercise during a fast.
◆ You should NOT do any exercise that is muscle building during a fast.
◆ You should not do any strenuous exercising during a fast. Strenuous is relative. A two mile jog is very light and easy to me, I can easily jog a mile or two per day during my fast but that may be very strenuous to some.
◆ You should keep warm while exercising.
◆ Walking and stretching are best.
◆ Fasting is NOT the time to GET IN SHAPE. Use exercise only to keep things moving and circulating.

Q: I get light headed or dizzy when I suddenly stand up or sit up, why?

A: This often occurs while fasting. The blood pressure is lowered during a fast and causes this effect. This is especially true during the heavy detox stages. You should get up slowly whenever you are rising from a sitting or prone position.

Q: Can I continue to go to work during a fast?

A: Most things with fasting depend on the factors involved. How long will you fast? What type of work do you do? What is your reason for fasting?

If your reason for fasting is a spiritual one, it is usually a good idea to isolate yourself from your daily routine activities and all negative influences. No TV, no movies and the music you listen to should reflect your spiritual values, etc.

If your work is pleasant, not stressful, and you enjoy the work and the people, then under most conditions, it is fine to go to work, during a short fast.

For a long fast, work is usually not a good idea. Your energy level can drop so low that you will not be very productive and you need to relax during that time. A short fast of one to three days with a NOT VERY TOXIC body will not usually present a problem.

If your body is very toxic, do not go to work at all. Plan your fast when you can either remain at home or get away to quiet and peaceful surroundings for a few days.

Q: Am I too skinny to fast?

A: **Why are you skinny?** As long as you are not skinny because you are starving or have an anorexia nervosa syndrome, it's fine for you to fast. It is generally true that a person with excess weight can survive without food longer than a skinny person. The skinny person's body may have fewer toxins, but the FAST FLUSH could create serious problems for the fat and the skinny person if they both suddenly stopped eating.

Skinny is also a relative term. Marilyn Monroe and Mae West were pin up girls and sex symbols during the height of their fame. By today's standards, they would be considered overweight for a movie star. In many cultures the standard of beauty is skinny by our standards. America is fat. We are unhealthy and overweight. Therefore if the average American is overweight, our idea of "skinny" is probably inflated.

As I mentioned previously, it is time for a fast to end when the body stops feeding upon toxins and diseased tissue and starts utilizing healthy tissue and technically moves into a state of starvation. As long as you stop a fast before that point, your body weight does not really matter.

Q: Can fasting hurt or injure me?

A: Yes! Just as any medicine can hurt or injure you, so can fasting if it is not done properly. Some people drop dead while jogging or playing basketball or having sex. Are any of these bad for you? Not generally, but problems can occur. Fasting puts a strain on the body. The serious cleaning that occurs can get rough. Just as the surgeon's knife can get rough.

The greater the level of toxicity or the greater the level of latent defects in your body, the greater the risk. That is true not just with fasting, but with anything. Fasting is not different from any other exercise or getting in shape process. It has certain risks.

Even walking has certain risks. People have heart attacks walking up stairs. Fasting can be a strain and usually is. You can minimize the risks, but you cannot eliminate them. QUICK FASTING is about making fasting as safe and as pleasant as possible. It is not about guaranteeing that nothing bad will ever happen. If you find something that guarantees that, please let me know right away.

Even the spiritual search has its physical risks. More people have been killed because of how they worship (religious conflicts, wars, and purgings) than any other cause. Everything has its risks, but certain risks are worth the reward. Fasting is one of those.

Q: *Am I too fat to fast? (See Chapter 19)*

A: Absolutely not! It may seem that the fatter you are, the longer you can fast. That is not necessarily true. It is true that excess body fat is an energy source. Excess body weight usually means excess toxins. Someone with a 50 pound potbelly is likely to be far more toxic than a slender person.

The toxins being removed could create major problems if the fast is not done correctly. You are not too fat to fast, but if your body is extremely toxic, and there is a good probability that it is, you must be very careful.

Chapter 16

SEX DURING FASTING

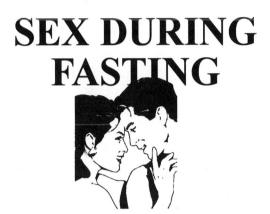

When I told my wife that I was going on a long fast, the first question she asked was, **"ARE WE GOING TO "DO IT" WHILE YOU ARE ON YOUR FAST?"**

There is rarely any advice given to the faster concerning sex. Many people need tons of advice about sex even if they aren't fasting, but if you're interested in sex, that's another book of mine called, <u>OH GOD! SEX FEELS GOOD–The Straight Talk Guide To Christian Sex</u> ISBN# 0-9631075-7-7

You must understand how sex works on the body, mind and spirit to understand its application during fasting. Sex has several major components to it.

- ◆ Sex Feels Good
- ◆ Sex is Emotional
- ◆ Sex is Good Exercise
- ◆ Sex is Spiritual
- ◆ Sex Changes Energy Levels
- ◆ Sex Changes Tension Levels

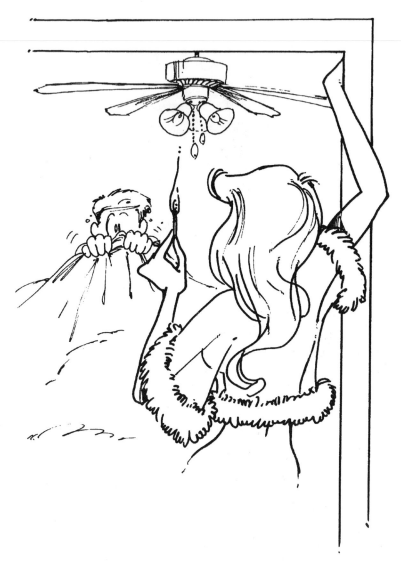

I know you're on a fast, but what about a little fast sex

◆ Sex Varies

Sex feels good. There is usually no argument about that even though the statement is not true for everyone. Some people get no enjoyment from sex. It is a chore and a dread for some. But for the vast majority of all creation with sex organs, sex is pleasurable.

Because sex feels good (and in some cases sex feels extremely good), this may be a prime reason for your sexual behavior during a fast. If you are married, there should be mutual consent if abstaining from sex during a fast. It is difficult to stop something that feels very good. If we did not get such a pleasure out of eating, most people would not become fat.

Sex is emotional. Sex usually generates strong emotional feelings over time. Women usually are more emotionally responsive initially, but I believe men get more attached in a good relationship in the long run.

Sex can bring out many different emotions, everything from love to extreme jealousy, from a great appreciation of a person to a great resentment. It can provoke feelings of unselfishness or an "out for self only" attitude. The emotion varies with the relationship, but one thing is certain. With time, sex will definitely change emotions.

Sex is good exercise. Depending upon how long and how vigorous sex is, it can be a very good exercise. If sex only lasts two or three minutes and you could put a dozen eggs under the couple without any of them breaking, chances are not much exercise is going on.

If on the other hand, the mattress wears out every couple of years, the couple gets up covered with sweat, and you miss an entire movie on television because you were sexually engaged, that is good exercise. Vigorous sex is aerobic and conditions the entire body.

One particular area that vigorous sex conditions is the abdomen region. The constant pelvic thrusting works the entire region from the upper thigh to below the breast bone. A major contributor to constipation and the clogging of the digestive system is a loose and flabby tone of the muscular system. Bowel movements improve when your abdomen is in shape. Good sex helps to get that region in condition.

Sex is spiritual. This book is not about my particular spiritual beliefs. All religions have laws concerning sexual behavior. All of the laws fundamentally boil down to this: **Whomever you have sex with, you should stay with.** By "stay with" I do not mean shack up together, but you should never break the relationship. In this society, it's called "marriage".

In the Old Testament of the Bible polygamy was allowed, but the principle of staying together was not violated. Even if a man had 10 wives, when he had sex with her, he stayed with her, and she with him.

There is a bond formed when sex occurs. A transfer of biological pheromones, hormones, essences, energies and other things we have yet to scientifically measure occurs. This effect is, of course, stronger between some than others, but there is an unseen, unmeasured effect that occurs when two human bodies sexually join.

Sex changes energy levels. After you have sex, I can guarantee you that your energy level will not be the same. You may feel energized or drained, but you will not feel the same. The second law of thermodynamics in essence states that, "when a system of higher energy comes in contact with a system of lower energy, the ENERGY ALWAYS flows from the higher source to the lower."

If a hot object touches a warm object, energy (heat) will flow from the hot object to the warm and never from the warm object to the hot. The human body is full of electrical impulses. It is like a giant wet cell battery. Electricity and other forms of energy flow simply from a touch. Sex is the most intimate and thorough, and wet, of the human touches. Energy flows one way or the other between the two bodies.

Energy also flows with the liquids that are discharged during sex, particularly for a man. The average male ejaculation contains 300 million sperm. That is enough sperm to repopulate the United States in every ejaculation. Those sperm are living, wiggling, swimming creatures.

Just as the principle, "to make something clean you must make something dirtier" exists, so do other principles. For something to live, something else must die.

For you to live, something else must die.

For you to live, something else must die. You eat a cow, or a chicken or a fish to live. The animal must die. You may be a vegetarian. I am 95% vegetarian yet for me to live, fruits must die, vegetables must die and nuts must die. All animals live from the death of other animals or plants.

Even plants live from the death of the sun. The sun is a massive fusion reactor that is slowly dying from using up its fuel. It may take a few million years, but it is dying. From its death, comes life.

Where do you think the life of those 300 million sperm comes from?

Ask most men how do they feel after sex, energized or sleepy? The vast majority will tell you that they feel sleepy. A life force or energy has left them when they ejaculate. The better condition the man is in, the less he will feel this effect but it occurs nonetheless.

Sex usually decreases a man's energy level after ejaculation. The woman often is not affected from a major drop in energy level.

Sex changes tension levels. Sex usually decreases tension. Particularly if it is very good. Sleepiness can result from a release of tension and not a decrease in energy level. During orgasm, the body tenses then relaxes. Even the orgasmic contractions are a series of hard contractions followed by relaxation, then contraction, then relaxation.

Sex reduces tension. If the sex is not under ideal conditions, it can increase tension. Pregnancy, AIDS, disease, infidelity and a host of other things can increase worry and tension after the short term release of sex. Sex changes tension levels. It immediately reduces tension in the physical, and may reduce or INCREASE it in the psychological which then affects the physical.

Sex varies. Sex varies depending on the couple and on the various times with the couple. Just as all loves are not created equal (at least among humans), neither are all sexual experiences. Sex can sometimes drain you to the point that you want to sleep all day. It can energize you to the point of wanting to stay up all night. Sex varies.

With these observations established, let's talk about sex and fasting.

Your sexual behavior during a fast depends upon several factors.

◆ **Why are you fasting?** Is it for health, weight loss or spiritual reasons.

◆ **How long are you fasting?** Is it one or two days or one or two weeks?

◆ **Are you a man or a woman?** Yes, it does make a difference when you are fasting.
◆ **Your sexual control?** I will explain that one shortly.

Sex is pleasurable. Most would like to continue to have sex during a fast. The only reason that we would not is if it was unhealthy, dangerous, or spiritually against what we wanted to do.

In the beginning stages of a fast, your energy will usually drop to a very low level. When your energy drops to a very low level, sex is the last thing on your mind. You can hardly get up much less get anything else up. The motivation and desire for sex is greatly diminished when your energy falls.

After the low energy period passes, sex pops back on your mind. Then what?

If you are fasting for spiritual reasons, you should avoid sex during your fast. Fasting from a spiritual perspective involves removing oneself from the carnal things of this world. Food is the most carnal thing. Yes, food is a greater carnal temptation than sex. Go seven days without sex, and then seven days without food and see which is harder. I used to think that sex was the greatest of the carnal temptations. That was before I fasted. Food is the strongest of the fleshly drives.

As I have said, the first thing we need is the warmth and touch of our mother's arms. Then we need food. Next comes the need for recognition, attention, THE EGO. The sex drive does not even develop until we are teenagers. It is the last drive to come in and the first drive to go out. It is with us for the shortest amount of time.

Fasting for spiritual purposes usually involves sacrificing

those things of the flesh and consecrating oneself to God. Many religious orders prohibit sex among those that have fully consecrated themselves to God. Many monastic orders, priests, nuns, and yogis completely give up sex.

For spiritual purposes, it is best to abstain from sex during your fast. You should have the consent and support of your spouse before doing this. It must be mutually agreed upon. If your wife or husband wants sex while you fast, your first obligation is to them. You need to be on one accord with your spouse.

Some religions that have ritual fasting, Islam for example, does not allow sex during the fasting period. Christianity has no definitive rules concerning what to do about sex during fasting. Be sure to read the rest of the advice about sex and fasting if you decide to have sex during your spiritual fast.

If you are fasting for weight loss or health reasons then the three other questions raised in the "it depends upon" section need to be answered.

How long are you fasting? If you are only fasting one to three days, having sex will not make a difference other than making you hungrier. During a fast the greatest hunger occurs during the first three days. After three days, hunger usually diminishes.

In general, I would recommend abstaining from sex if you are fasting. For a short 1-3 day fast, even though sex will make you hungrier, it should not harm you. The pelvic thrusting may actually help the intestines to clear the accumulated material from your system.

Sex during ANY fast is NOT THE BEST IDEA. The best idea is to have sex during your pre-fast regime on The Eden Diet and to abstain from sex during your fast.

If you are planning on a longer fast, over three days,

it is best to abstain from sex. The energy drain may get too rough, especially for a man. If you can't abstain, for reasons of either discipline or lack of spousal support, then at least follow certain guidelines.

Are you a man or woman? In case you have not noticed, the sexual organs of a man are different than those of a woman. Therefore, the sexual arousal, response, orgasm, recovery and ejaculation are also different between the sexes. If you are a woman, then my advice concerning sex and fasting is different.

When you have sex with your spouse, do you feel refreshed and energized or drained? Persons can have totally opposite aftermath sexual responses. If you feel refreshed and energized, then the sexual experience is providing you with energy. If you feel drained afterwards, then it is draining you of energy.

If you are an energy recipient, then obviously, sex during the fast will not drain your energy (beyond the exercise factor) to have sex. If you are an energy donor, or you feel drained, I would strongly advise against having sex during a fast. As I mentioned, sex varies. That ends my sexual advice to women. In summary, it is better if you abstain. It is not so bad if you are being energized, but it will severely deplete your energy if you are being drained during sex.

If you are a man then the last question applies only to you. How is your sexual control?

Ejaculation is universally draining for a man. I don't care who you are, ejaculation will drain you of your life force and energy. If you are in great shape or very young, the drain may be almost unnoticeable, but the drain is there. Three hundred million living sperm leave a man's body swimming in a nutrient rich stream. Your body has to draw upon its resources to replenish them and that drains you.

If you must have sex
DO NOT EJACULATE!!!

To learn to control this is not easy. If you do not ejaculate, you will not lose the energy. You will only exercise. This may even improve your sex life after the fast as it will help you learn to control ejaculation. A significant percentage of the male population has a problem with that.

There are techniques to train a man how to have sex and have an orgasm and no ejaculation, but that's another book. When you master that, you will gain more discipline than just food control.

Chapter 17

COVERING THE OTHER HOLES OF THE BODY

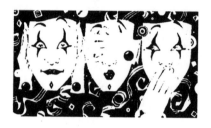

During a fast, particularly a spiritual fast, it is important not just to abstain from food(s), but to undergo a period of physical, mental and spiritual cleansing.

There is a reason the spiritual masters wanted to be alone when they fasted. Because even in the ancient days, most of what they saw and heard among the people of the city was negative.

The human body has nine holes in it, (yes, count them). It is no coincidence that you play two nine hole rounds of golf. When you combine two people, you have 18 holes, when you play the front and back nine in golf, you play 18 holes. Haven't you ever wondered where they got 18 holes from?

Two eyes, two ears, two nostrils and a mouth make seven holes in the head. For a man, the anus and the penile urethral opening make nine. For a woman the anus and the vagina

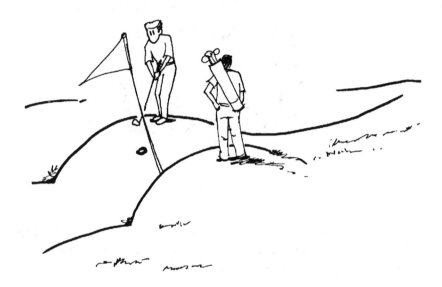

The human body has nine holes in it, (yes, count them). It is no coincidence that you play two nine hole rounds of golf. When you combine two people, you have 18 holes, when you play the front and back nine in golf, you play 18 holes. Haven't you ever wondered where they got 18 holes from?

make nine. Technically, the woman also has a urethral opening, which makes the vagina the tenth hole. Have you ever wondered why men call the golf club house the 19th hole? Where they celebrate and drink? Just a thought.

During a fast, it is important to pay careful attention to all the holes. We have discussed the anus, (cleaning the colon and intestines), we have discussed the urethral opening, (drinking plenty of water to flush the system) and sex. We have discussed the vagina, (sex again).

The other holes of the body are just as important. For the spiritual fast, they are of utmost importance. When you stop eating, something happens to your mind and spirit.

The mind and spirit go through an initial period of turmoil as the body is cleaned out. Then the mind becomes peaceful.

It rises above mundane things of the world. You will be surprised how many things lose their importance when you stop eating for a period of time.

When the body is clean, it becomes like a sponge. A clean rag will take up dirt faster than a dirty one. When the mind is clean, it also becomes like a sponge. Guard your holes. When fasting, avoid watching television.

Ninety percent of the things on TV are negative. Soap operas, violent TV shows, distressing situations, twisted relationships and talk shows that address the weirdest, most perverted things that you can imagine are what dominate the television airwaves. Then there is the news.

Every horrible murder, rape, robbery, corruption, war and conceivable atrocity is distilled from around your city, state, America and the world. They are then concentrated and dropped into your den, living room or bedroom to pour into the waiting holes of your eyes and ears.

You are not just what you eat, but you are what you take

in through ALL of your holes. What you take in will be reflected in what you let out. Just as an animal's diet can be analyzed by its feces, so can yours. Do you know how much can be told about your health and what is in your system just from a urine sample?

There are five holes in the body that things come out of on a regular basis: the anus, the urethral opening, the nostrils and the mouth. What you speak is influenced by what goes into the holes in your head. If you watch constant violence, conflict, wars and twisted relationships on television what comes out of your mouth will reflect what went into your eyes and ears.

You will speak fear, hate, skepticism, doubt for the future, and trouble into your own life because you have allowed mess to enter into the holes in your head. Guard ALL of your holes. This is not just true during a fast, it is true continually and it is vitally important during a fast. Turn off the television, turn off the radio, do not read the newspaper (it is also mostly negative news), stay away from ALL negative influences during your fast. The same advice applies to movies.

If you read, read only those things that will assist you in your spiritual rise. If you must watch television, carefully screen your programs (in advance) to watch only those programs that will help you in your spiritual quest. Remember, television programs are LOADED with FOOD commercials (mostly unhealthy). DO NOT expose yourself to temptation!

Finally, brethren, whatsoever things are true, whatsoever things are honest, whatsoever things are just, whatsoever things are pure, whatsoever things are lovely, whatsoever things are of good report; if there be any virtue, and if there be any praise, think on these things. Phil 4:8

Chapter 18

HOW TO BREAK YOUR FAST

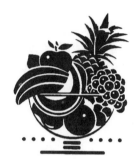

The word BREAKFAST means to break your fast. We do it each morning after our bodies have undergone a mini-fast during the night.

BREAKING A FAST PROPERLY IS JUST AS IMPORTANT AS THE PRE-FAST PROGRAM AND WHAT YOU DO ON THE FAST!!!

Two of the greatest mistakes of the uninformed are eating a huge, hard to digest meal before they fast, and eating a huge, hard to digest meal when they break a fast.

I have heard many people say, "I am preparing to go on a fast, so I am going to go out and eat a big steak dinner as my last meal." That big improperly combined steak, bread and potato dinner sits and rots in the digestive system during the entire fast.

The next statement is, "I have just finished fasting for seven days, I'm going out to the same restaurant where I had the big steak dinner as my last meal and get another one as my first meal."

Eating the wrong meal after a fast can literally turn a first meal into a last meal. When on a long fast, five days or more, the digestive system shuts down partially or completely. All energy is redirected. If you have cleaned out well, the stomach and the intestines are clean.

The system is not only cleaned of toxins, but it also cleans out the intestinal flora. Certain "good" bacteria live in your digestive tract (the intestinal flora). A thorough fast cleans out everything. You must allow time for the digestive system to prepare itself for food again.

How you should break your fast depends upon how long you have fasted. A good rule to follow is one day of a special diet for each five days that you fast and your first meal after any fast should not be a heavy full meal.

The special diet should only consist of dead fruit juices or herbal teas. When I say "dead fruit juices," I mean juices that are bottled or either fresh juices that you have heated to kill the enzymes. The reason for this is to prevent the active enzymes in the fresh juices from becoming a shock to the system. Bottled fruit juice is usually pasteurized, therefore, the enzymes in them are deactivated. Buy only non-sugared fruit juice that is pure fruit juice. Do not buy fruit drinks with sugar or other sweeteners.

It is best to squeeze and heat your own juices. Simmer the juices for 5 to 10 minutes, then allow them to cool to room temperature. It is best to eat everything during the BREAK FAST period at room temperature, nothing cold and nothing hot.

Acid fruits, such as oranges and grapefruits are best. Grapes are also good. Natural bottled apple juice and grape juice are easy to find at any grocery store.

This only applies to fasts of five days or longer. A shorter fast will generally not destroy the bacteria or shut down the digestive system.

A good rule of thumb for a short fast is to eat **ONE FRESH FRUIT MEAL FOR EACH DAY OF YOUR FAST.** If you fast for three days, then your first three meals should be fresh fruit. Even a one day fast should be broken with only fresh fruit. Many toxins and solid wastes will be loosened during a short fast. Fresh fruit is the best way to get them out of the body.

If you eat solid food after a long fast, the first thing that will occur is constipation. Your digestive system will not move that solid food until it starts functioning again. It has been busy cleaning, not digesting.

How you break your fast has a major effect on the benefits that you receive from your fast.

If you eat dairy products, plain yogurt is also good after the fruit juices. Yogurt contains "good" bacteria that help to restore the intestinal flora.

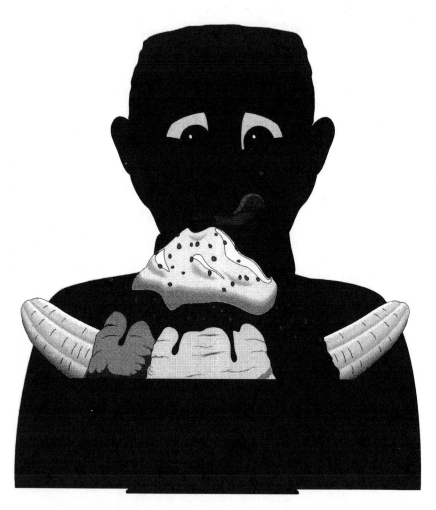

The number of seriously overweight Americans jumped to 33% (an increase of over 30%) during the 1980s and 90s. The figures show an even more dangerous trend in the younger generation.

Chapter 19

FASTING
TO LOSE WEIGHT

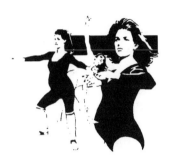

A long term study by the federal Centers for Disease Control and Prevention shocked scientists. The study showed that 1/4 (25%) of Americans were seriously overweight in the 1960s and 70s.

The number of seriously overweight Americans jumped to 33% (an increase of over 30%), during the 1980s and 90s. The figures show an even more dangerous trend in the younger generation. 15 percent of teenagers were seriously overweight in the 1970s. In 1991, the figure was 21 percent, a 40 percent increase in fat teenagers. Usually, most people don't get fat until they become adults.

The average child watches 10,000 TV commercials a year advertising food. The commercials are not advertising fruit and broccoli either.

They are watching pizza commercials with rubbery, sticky, cheese that behaves like a very strong rubber band (and we wonder why constipation is so high). Can you imagine that cheese trying to get through your stomach and intestines? They are watching hamburger commercials with two, three or four fried greasy patties, greasy bacon piled on, greasy sauce, served with a super large order of greasy fries, washed down with a gigantic sugary drink. They are watching candy commercials with cute talking candy pieces and breakfast cereals that contain up to 50% sugar.

Even the portions of the food have drastically gone up. A large order of french fries is a meal (although an unhealthy one) in itself. You can order soft drinks that are 64 oz., that's two quarts of sugary drink for one person. And we wonder why we are getting fatter. In addition, the cost of junk food has gone way down. A hamburger and fries are cheaper now than they were 10 years ago.

You can buy a large double patty burger cheap. A meal from a fast food restaurant, large burger, large fries, and large drink costs less than a wholesome meal prepared at home. Junk food has become cheap, and health care has become expensive. You pay on one end or the other.

Why are we so fat? We are being advertised to, cajoled, tempted and then given super fattening food to satisfy our desires. Social conditions even play a part.

The CDC study found the highest rate of obesity, up to 70%, among some Native American (American Indian) groups. Next in line were Black and Mexican-American women, with nearly 50% of the adult women fat. White women had a rate of 33.5% fat.

In 1965, a study showed that the rate of obesity among the poorest groups of people was five times as great as among the richest. America has a backwards fat rate.

In some cultures, it is the rich people who are fat and the poor people who are thin. In America the rich are thin and the poor are fat. Being fat as a sign of prosperity still exists in some cultures of the world.

In those cultures, it is understandable. Food is money and having food is a sign of having money. In the Bible when a depression hit the land, they called it a famine and their major concern was food. In America, we are concerned about many things, but starving is not one of them. You can go to the poorest of any American community, white or black, and you will see a large amount of people that are grossly overweight. There may be a shortage of proper nutrition, but there is no shortage of food.

The pressures of life undoubtedly pile up higher on the lower socioeconomic end. Food has always been an outlet, almost like a drug. Much obesity is traceable to depression. When we feel bad, or alone, or unloved, or abused, or discriminated against, or powerless or poor, we often eat to ease the pain.

But fatness in America ultimately has its roots in our inability to control our flesh. And it's getting worse. This nation needs control. This nation, like the ancient ones, needs to fast.

The waistlines are steadily moving up. America is getting fatter and fatter, among the young and the not so young. The technical term is "obese" but I will cut through the politically correct word and call things as they are. America is getting fatter.

America has a weight problem. More precisely, an eating problem that manifests itself as a weight problem. That's a critical point to understand. **The problem is not the weight.** The weight is the result or the fruit of the problem. The problem is:

WE CANNOT CONTROL OUR APPETITE.

If we control the appetite, the weight is automatically controlled. I am not talking about the small percentage of

Americans that have a glandular problem. I am speaking about the vast majority of us that cannot control our diet.

When thou sittest to eat with a ruler, consider diligently what is before thee: And put a knife to thy throat, if thou be a man given to appetite. Prov 23:1-2

The NIV translation puts it this way:

When you sit to dine with a ruler, note well what is before you, and put a knife to your throat if you are given to gluttony.

When we cannot control our appetite, we literally are putting a knife to our throats (the ancient symbolism for killing yourself). Being fat puts you at a greatly increased risk of heart attacks, strokes, diabetes, gout, arthritis, many forms of cancer and a host of other ailments. The knife at our throats may be a surgeon's knife on the operating table.

We are trying to diet, but failing miserably. Only 5% of people who go on a diet and lose weight keep the weight off for five years. What happens to the other 95%? They remain fat or get fatter.

Is it that the diets don't work? Yes, and no. . . The diets work, we don't. We lack the discipline to control our diets and eventually slip back to old habit patterns.

There was plenty of dieting in the Bible. It was called fasting. Fasting is simply the restriction of our usual eating. Whether a fruit fast or a water fast or a fast from meat, or beef or sweets, fasting is a restriction of our food, a diet.

People have had the same temptations and weaknesses throughout recorded history. I do not see that changing any time soon. Food has always been one of those weaknesses. Fasting is a way to overcome the food weakness.

Fasting can be a real life saver for the overweight person. The benefit of fasting is not in weight loss. Fasting will make you lose weight. A water fast will result in an average of 1 to 2 pounds per day of weight loss. But that is not the benefit of fasting for weight loss.

"I think that will benefit me," you may say, especially if you are overweight. But that is not the total truth of fasting and weight loss.

Fasting can actually make you fatter.

The power of fasting is not in losing weight during the fast, but in gaining control of your appetite, which is the REAL problem.

During a fast, the body burns its own fat. As the body burns its fat there is a release of chemical compounds called "ketones". Medical science claims this is the source of "bad breath." That is partially true. I am familiar with the smell of ketones from my chemistry training. When ketones are released, I did smell them, but the other stuff that was on my breath was NOT KETONES. The stuff that came out in the enema was NOT KETONES, it was M.E.S.S..

As the body burns fat, eliminates M.E.S.S. and cleanses itself, two things happen that can make you fatter.

First, after several days, your metabolism slows down. If your body were being described as a car, metabolism would be all of the engine and battery processes. The body slows its metabolism approximately 20% after several days on a fast. Medical science describes this as a survival mechanism.

If the body is not getting food, then it slows down so that it needs less food, that makes plenty sense. This way, you can live much longer with no food if your body slows down.

Second, your digestive system is cleaner. The villi in the intestines are cleaner, the stomach lining is cleaner, the colon is cleaner.

When a car engine gets dirty, it uses more gas per mile. If the spark plugs are dirty, the carburetor or fuel injectors clogged, the wires corroded, and the air filter is clogged, the engine does not run efficiently.

Clean up the car engine and your gas mileage will improve. You can go farther from the same gallon of gas. The same is true of your body.

If the lungs are clogged, the intestines coated with filth, the colon stopped up, the blood thick and sluggish, fat surrounding the heart and in the arteries, the body is running inefficiently. Clean up the body, and you will get more miles to the gallon.

A fast cleans up the body.
A fast slows the metabolism.

When you combine those two elements, a cleaner more efficient body with a slower metabolism, you need less food for the same level of activity. Food is absorbed and utilized better in a clean digestive system. It does not take a research team to spend years testing, analyzing, taking surveys and doing clinical trials to prove that. That is common sense.

If it takes less food to do the same thing, it means one of three things:

1. You need to cut down on the food you were eating before the fast since you do not need as much food for the same level of activity.

2. If you eat the same amount of food after the fast as before, you need more physical activity to use the extra efficiency and slowed metabolism.

3. If you eat the same, and have the same activity level, you may get fatter!

I am trying to tell you the truth as I understand it. I will not lie or make fasting sound like something it is not.

Fasting can make you fatter if you don't change after the fast.

Fasting will allow you to gain control of your appetite. There comes a power of self-control after you have completed a long fast that is like nothing else. You may not get the self-control that you seek on your first fast. But, do you master anything else on your first try?

Fasting on a periodic basis allows a person to gradually gain control over their appetite. Do not gorge before or after the fast! Learning to control your desire for food as you break your fast is a great aid in controlling it daily.

You will find that you are not hungry when you end your fast (after three days, hunger usually abates). You are not hungry, but the desire to eat is there. There is a big difference between actual hunger and desire for food.

Learn to control the desire, learn to eat only when you are physically hungry. **This is the ONLY way any type of permanent weight loss becomes effective.** You must have a change of thought pattern and a change of lifestyle.

A diet is always viewed as a punishment. We don't like punishment. I don't care who you are, eventually you will move away from punishment to that which is rewarding.

The only way to successfully lose weight is to CHANGE what we view as rewarding. As long as stuffing yourself with food, eating three or more clogging meals per day and sweets and fattening foods are your idea of reward, you will remain either fat or on a constant weight yo-yo.

READ the book *FIT FOR LIFE*. I highly recommend it. It has practical solutions and easy to understand explanations of why and what you should do to keep your weight at the level you desire.

      Fasting will make you lose weight, but only a change of lifestyle and MENTALITY will make you keep it off.

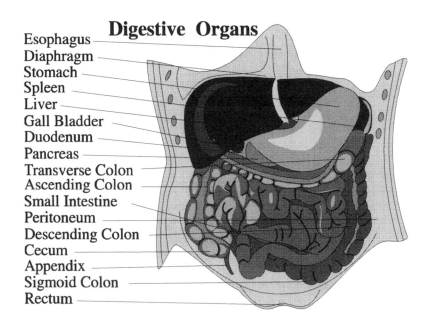

Digestive Organs

Esophagus
Diaphragm
Stomach
Spleen
Liver
Gall Bladder
Duodenum
Pancreas
Transverse Colon
Ascending Colon
Small Intestine
Peritoneum
Descending Colon
Cecum
Appendix
Sigmoid Colon
Rectum

Chapter 20

WARNING TO FASTERS WITH ILLNESSES

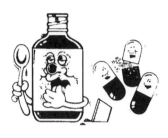

If you have a major illness such as diabetes, kidney problems, liver problems, heart problems or ulcers, do not fast without consulting a professional. Be sure to read the chapter, "Consulting A Doctor."

Fasting puts the body under a strain. The liver and kidney are organs of purification and elimination that will go into overtime during a fast. Blood sugar levels change drastically as stored glycogen is converted into glucose (blood sugar) for use by the body. That can be extremely risky for a diabetic. The toxic shock of poisons being eliminated can literally stop a weak heart.

Although I believe fasting is a divine, correct and beneficial venture, the more we have abused our bodies and the worse condition it is in, the more taxing the fast will be.

Always seek professional advice if you are on any medication.

How to properly BM.

I can hear you saying, "I may not know a lot about fasting, but I know how to BM. I have been BMing all of my life." I know you have been BMing all of your life, but you probably have not been BMing properly.

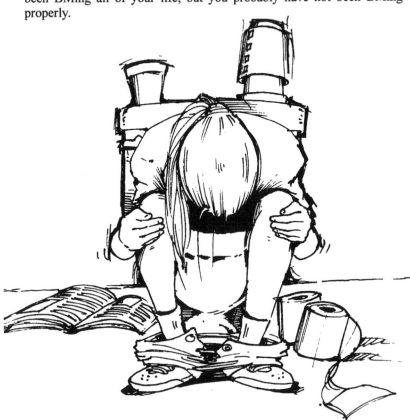

How can you squat on a commode?

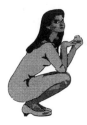
You can't practically, but you can imitate the same relative positioning and muscle tension as squatting.
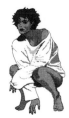

Chapter 21

REGULAR SCHEDULED FASTING

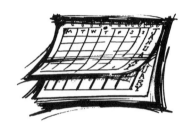

I would recommend that everyone (who can) fast on a regular basis. Once the body is clean, a periodic maintenance fast allows the body to both rest and clean itself.

My recommendation for the new faster is as follows:

Experienced fasters may fast longer and more regularly but this is a practical program that most people can follow.

Once Per Year — A 7 Day Fast.

This should be done at a particular time each year to keep it on schedule. You may want to start on New Year's Day or the day after your birthday. Fasts are better adhered to when there is a set date each year for you to begin.

The 7 day water fast should be preceded by a 7 day Eden Diet for a total of 14 days of cleansing. The 7 days of water should coincide with a period when you do not have to work.

These 14 days each year will allow you to renew and refresh your body.

40 Hours — Once Per Week

Again, a regular time each week must be established for the discipline to be maintained. Your spouse needs to fast along with you. It makes things far more difficult if one person in the household is eating and another is fasting.

For the 40-hour weekly fast, eat only the Eden Diet one day until 3p.m. Fast on water the next day, then break fast with fresh fruit at 7 a.m. the next morning.

For example, if Tuesday is your chosen day:

Monday - The Eden Diet until 3 p.m.- 4 p.m.

Tuesday - Distilled Water

Wednesday - 7 a.m. - 8 a.m. Fresh Fruit meal

Your 40 hours would end at 7 a.m. or 8 a.m. depending on whether you stopped eating at 3 p.m. or 4 p.m.

Your fasting schedule can be tailored to suit your needs and discipline level. You may have to start with an 8 hour fast, or a fast of just one meal a day.

As you learn to control your food, you will learn to control other things about yourself. As you become master over one thing, it will lead to mastery over many.

Fasting works, but only if you do. It is not easy in the beginning, but nothing worthwhile ever is. It takes energy and effort to change. It takes energy and effort to change for the better, change for the worse is easy. To change for the worst, you only need to follow the crowd, that path is always wide and well traveled. May your path be narrow.

Fasting will help you to change for the better.

I wish you well,

and whether you believe as I do or not. . .

God Bless You

Bowles, Willa Vae, **Fasting For A Modern Day Lifestyle,** *Total Health,* Oct 1988 v10 n5 p45

Morris, Lois B., **Escape From Excess: an over-stuffer learns to eat...when she's hungry,** *Health,* May 1990, v22 n5 p58

Braverman, Eric R., **Emotions and the Nazarite Diet,** *Total Health,* Feb 1989, v11 p8

Diet and Rheumatoid Arthritis: **new study shows benefit-fasting and vegetarianism improve symptoms,** *HealthFacts,* Nov. 1991, v16 n150 p3

Baker, Elizabeth, Cleansing Diets: **How to Avoid Colds and Flu,** *Total Health,* Feb 1989, v11 p47

Newman, Jennifer, **The Joys of Eating Alone,** *American Health,* Dec. 1989, v8 n10 p82

Hyman, Jane Wegscheider, **You Are When You Eat,** *East West,* Aug. 1990 v20 n8 p46

Omartian, Stormie, **Seven Steps to Greater Health, Youthfulness and Vitality,** *Total Health,* Feb 1989, v11 n1 p17

Jennings-Sauer, Cheryl, **What Have You Got to Lose-Medically Supervised Fasts,** *American Health,* Mar 1989 v8 n2 p155

Duhamel, Denise, **Holding Fast,** *American Health,* May 1990, v9 n4 p44

Cross, J.H.: Eminson, J.; Warton, B.A., **Ramadan and Birth Weight at Full Term in Asian Moslem Pregnant Women in Birmingham,** *Archives of Disease in Childhood,* Oct 1990 v65 n10 p1053

Success On Very Low Calorie Diets, *Nutrition Research Newsletter,* July-August 1991, v10 n7-8 p78

Graham, Janis, **Is Fasting Worth It?,** *Health,* July-August 1991, v23 n6 p46

Thompson, Tricia, **The Hungry High (The Fasting Controversy),** *Harper's Bazaar,* Jan 1992 v125 n3361 p80

Insights Into Fasting, *The Lancet,* Jan 10, 1992 v339 n8786 p152

Rashed, Awad H., **The Fast of Ramadan: No Problems for the Well: The Sick Should Avoid Fasting,** *British Medical Journal,* Feb 1992, v304 n6826 p521

Braverman, Eric, **The Benefits of Fasting,** *Total Health,* June 1994 v16 n3 p46

Vegetable Juices Have Many Worthy Nutrients, *Better Nutrition for Today's Living,* Nov. 1994 v56 n11 p22

McCarthy, Laura Flynn, **Liquid Lessons (liquid diets),** *Harper's Bazaar,* Jan 1992 v125 n3361 p81

Partee, Phillip, **The Layman's Guide to Fasting and Losing Weight,** *United Press,* Sarasota, Fl, 1979

Boswell, John, **Holy Feast and Holy Fast-The Religious Significance of Food to Medieval Women,** *The New Republic,* Aug. 24, 1987 v197 p36

Ehret, Arnold, **Rational Fasting,** *Ehret Publishing,* Beaumont CA, 1972

Ehret, Arnold, **The Mucusless Diet Healing System,** *Ehret Publishing,* Beaumont CA, 1975

Lawrence, Leslie, **Senseless Starvation,** *Harper's Bazaar,* Jan 1992, v125 n3361 p83

Freedman, Donna, **Why Are You Hungry?,** *Nation's Business,* May 1989, v77 n5 p69

Chilnick, Lawrence D., **The Pill Book,** *Bantam Books,* N.Y.,N.Y., 1990

Diamond, Harvey and Marilyn, **Fit For Life,** *Warner Books,* N.Y.,N.Y., 1985

Elmer-Dewitt, Philip, **Fat Times,** *Time,* Jan 16, 1995 v145 n2 p58

Long, James, W., **The Essential Guide To Prescription Drugs,** *Harper Collings,* N.Y.,N.Y., 1991

DeHaan, M.R., **The Chemistry of The Blood,** *Zondervan Publishing,* Grand Rapids, MI, 1981

Bragg, Paul and Patricia, **Bragg Toxicless Diet Body Purification and Healing System,** *Health Science,* Santa Barbara, CA

Jensen, Bernard, **Tissue Cleaning Through Bowel Management,** *Bernard Jensen Enterprises,* Escondido CA, 1981

O R D E R   F O R M

Bronner Books are available from Century Systems at quantity discount for ministries, institutions, schools, businesses, and other organizations. For more information, call or write to: Century Systems Inc., Box 43725, Atlanta, GA 30336 1-800-843-9662. You may send letters to the author at the above address, your letters will be forwarded.

Fax orders (404) 696-2480
Visa/MC/Amex orders (24hrs/day) call 1-800-843-9662
internet e-mail nbronner@1800thewoman.com
full text of books are online at www.1800thewoman.com
Check or Money Order orders mail to:
Century Systems, Box 43725, Atlanta, GA 30336

Please send me the following number of copies of Bronner books at 9.95 ea. plus 2.00 ea p&h:

Qty	Title	ISBN#
_____	**Get A Grip**	**0-9631075-2-6**
_____	**Just For The Asking**	**0-9631075-3-4**
_____	**Quick Fasting**	**0-9631075-1-8**
_____	**How To Find God**	**0-9631075-5-0**

Total Number of books _____   **x 9.95 ea. =** _____

Total Number of books _____   **x 2.00 p&h=** _____

☐**Ck/MO enclosed**   ☐ **Visa/MC**   **Total** _____

(Georgia residents add 7% tax)

Please RUSH my books to: (Please Print)

Name _____

Address _____

City_____ **State**_____ **Zip** _____

Visa/MC#_____ **Exp** _____

Signature _____

VISA/MC ORDERS CALL TOLL FREE 24 HOURS A DAY
1-800-THE-WOMAN   1-800-843-9662